Blood Collection

A SHORT COURSE

EDITION 2

Blood Collection
A SHORT COURSE

EDITION 2

Marjorie Schaub Di Lorenzo, MT(ASCP)SH
Adjunct Clinical Laboratory Science Instructor
Division of Clinical Laboratory Science
School of Allied Health Professions
University of Nebraska Medical Center
Omaha, Nebraska
Phlebotomy Technician Program Coordinator
Health Professions
Nebraska Methodist College – The Josie Harper Campus
Omaha, Nebraska

Susan King Strasinger, DA, MT(ASCP)
Faculty Associate
The University of West Florida
Pensacola, Florida

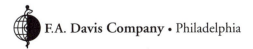

F.A. Davis Company • Philadelphia

F. A. Davis Company
1915 Arch Street
Philadelphia, PA 19103
www.fadavis.com

Copyright © 2010 by F. A. Davis Company

Printed in the United States of America

Last digit indicates print number: 10 9 8 7 6 5 4 3 2 1

Senior Acquisitions Editor: Christa Fratantoro
Manager of Content Development: George W. Lang
Developmental Editor: David Payne
Art and Design Manager: Carolyn O'Brien
Cover photo courtesy of photos.com

Library of Congress Cataloging-in-Publication Data
Di Lorenzo, Marjorie Schaub, 1953-
   Blood collection : a short course / Marjorie Schaub Di Lorenzo, Susan King Strasinger. — 2nd ed.
       p. ; cm.
   Rev. ed. of: Blood collection in healthcare / Marjorie Schaub Di Lorenzo, Susan King Strasinger. c2002.
   Includes bibliographical references and index.
   ISBN-13: 978-0-8036-1699-8
   ISBN-10: 0-8036-1699-6
   ISBN-10: (invalid) 0-8036-2056-X
  1. Blood—Collection and preservation. 2. Phlebotomy. I. Strasinger, Susan King. II. Di Lorenzo, Marjorie Schaub, 1953- Blood collection in healthcare. III. Title.
   [DNLM: 1. Phlebotomy—instrumentation. 2. Phlebotomy—methods. 3. Blood Specimen Collection—instrumentation. 4. Blood Specimen Collection—methods. QY 25 D525b 2009]
   RB45.15.D525 2009
   616.07'561—dc22

                                                                                          2009002932

To my husband, Scott,
and my children, Michael, Christopher, and Lauren
MSD

To Harry,
you will always be my Editor-in-Chief
SKS

Preface

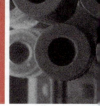

This short course textbook is designed to provide practicing health-care personnel with concise information on the proper techniques to collect quality blood specimens with minimal patient discomfort. The purpose of the book, *Blood Collection: A Short Course*, Edition 2, is primarily for the cross-training and continuing education of health-care professionals currently performing phlebotomy work or those who anticipate performing phlebotomy procedures in the future. Today's concept of developing health-care teams to help streamline patient care has evolved to encompass the cross-training of nurses, respiratory therapists, radiographers, medical assistants, certified nursing assistants, and medical technologists. Phlebotomy has become a major part of this cross-training.

Topics emphasized in the text include the following:

- Types of blood required for specific lab tests
- Purpose of these tests, vein selection, and alternate sites
- Types of collection tubes and the purpose of anticoagulants
- Order of draw
- Test-specific handling
- Complications and remedies
- Storage and transportation conditions

In addition, *Blood Collection*, Edition 2, includes two new chapters on point-of-care testing, and IVs and central venous access devices (CVADs). Information common to all health-care curriculums, such as safety precautions, anatomy and physiology, quality assurance, and patient-caregiver interactions, is covered only in the context of their relationship to the collection of blood specimens.

This current comprehensive text provides a cost-effective, compact learning tool for phlebotomy short courses. Coverage of the following topics is included in this edition:

- Blood collection equipment, including the newest safety devices
- Technical procedures for venipuncture and dermal puncture
- Special collection procedures, including access to central venous catheters and IV insertion and care
- Specimen handling, storage, and transport procedures
- Methods to increase the quality of blood specimens
- Correlation of laboratory tests and clinical disorders
- Quality assurance procedures required by laboratory regulatory agencies as they relate to phlebotomy

Note that all procedures are written to comply with the standards set forth by the Occupational Safety and Health Administration, The Joint Commission, and the Clinical and Laboratory Standards Institute.

Moreover, the following pedagogical features are included in this text to facilitate learning:

- **Learning objectives**
- **Technical tips**, to avoid complications, such as hematomas and hemolysis
- **Safety tips**
- **Practical situation problem-solving exercises**
- **Performance evaluation checklists** for technical procedures
- **Review questions**
- **Numerous illustrations, photographs, diagrams, charts, and tables**
- **Internet Help**

This text provides a quick reference with the most current updates for blood collection skills. Appendices list reference material, such as frequently ordered laboratory tests with the required types of anticoagulants and volume of blood required. A summary of laboratory tests, their functions, and their clinical correlation is included. Answer keys for the situation problem-solving exercises and review questions sections also are available. A complete color tube guide lists all the different types of collection tubes, the additives, number of inversions required, and laboratory uses of the tubes. A PowerPoint presentation, Lecture Outlines, and a Comprehensive Test with answers provide instructors who adopt the book with additional instructional tools.

We specifically designed this text to meet the needs of nurses and other health-care professionals who want and need to add a new phlebotomy competency or to reinforce past learned skills. It can be used to promote learning in academic settings, hospital-training sessions, or continuing education courses.

REFERENCES

Clinical and Laboratory Standards Institute. Procedures for the Collection of Diagnostic Blood Specimens by Venipuncture, ed. 6. Approved Standard, H3-A6, Wayne, PA, 2007.

Clinical and Laboratory Standards Institute. Procedures for the Handling and Processing of Blood Specimens, ed. 3. Approved Guideline, H18-A3, Wayne, PA, 2004.

Clinical and Laboratory Standards Institute. Procedures and Devices for the Collection of Diagnostic Capillary Blood Specimens, Approved Standard, ed. 6. H4-A6, Wayne, PA, 2008.

Clinical and Laboratory Standards Institute, Tubes and Additives for Venous Blood Specimen Collection, Approved Standard, ed. 5, Wayne, PA, 2003.

Elkin, Perry, & Potter, (2007). Nursing Intervention & Clinical Skills, 4th Edition. St. Louis, Missouri: Mosby, Inc.

Policies and Procedures for Infusion Nursing, 3rd Edition, pages 168–172. Infusion Nurses Society, 2006.

Strasinger, SK and Di Lorenzo, MS. The Phlebotomy Workbook, ed. 2. FA Davis, Philadelphia, 2003.

Contributors

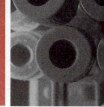

Brenda L. M. Franks, BS, MT(ASCP)
Point-of-Care Testing Coordinator
Nebraska Methodist Health System
Omaha, Nebraska
Unit 7: Point-of-Care Testing

Karen Maggio-LaRose, RN, MSN
Staff Nurse
Joint Ambulatory Care Center
Gulf Coast Veterans Health Care System
Pensacola, Florida
Unit 8: Intravenous Insertion and Central
Venous Catheter Assess

Reviewers

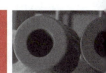

Karen Gordon, CLS(NCA), MT(ASCP)SLS, PBT(ASCP)
Clinical Education Coordinator
Phlebotomy
Northern Virginia University
Falls River, Virginia

Jeanne Griffith, BS
Director of Training
OIC Training Academy
Fairmont, West Virginia

Frankie Harris-Lyne, MLT (ASCP), CLS
Assistant Dean
Allied Health Division
Medical Laboratory Technology & Phlebotomy
Programs
Northern Virginia Community College
Springfield, Virginia

Brenna Ildza, MT (ASCP)SH, PBT
Director of Phlebotomy Education Program
Pathology Department
Saint Luke's Hospital
Kansas City, Missouri

Patty Janousek, BSN, CRNI
Methodist Hospital
IV Team Leader
Omaha, Nebraska

Mary Shivers
MLT Program Director
Copiah-Lincoln Community College
Wesson, Missouri

Diane Wolff, MLT(ASCP)
Methodist Hospital
Phlebotomy Team Leader
Omaha, Nebraska

Acknowledgments

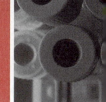

Many individuals gave of their time and expertise to make this 2nd edition of *Blood Collection: A Short Course* and the accompanying instructor CD-ROM possible. We wish to thank Diane Wolff, MLT (ASCP), Phlebotomy Team Leader, Brenda Franks, BS, MT(ASCP), POCT Coordinator, Patty Janousek, BSN,CRNI, IV Team Leader, and the administration and staff at Methodist Hospital for their continued support. We also wish to thank photographer Tim McCormick, Billings Photography, and the manufacturers who allowed us to illustrate their products. We thank Sherman Bonomelli, MS from the University of West Florida Clinical Laboratory Science Program for contributing visual concepts that became the foundation for many of the line illustrations. We are grateful for the dedication of the staff at F.A. Davis, especially those with whom we have worked most closely: David Payne, Developmental Editor, George Lang, Manager of Content Development, Elizabeth Stepchin, Developmental Associate, and Christa Fratantoro, Senior Acquisitions Editor.

Contents

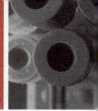

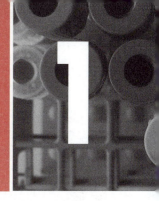

Introduction to Blood Collection

1

Introduction

The redesigning of the health-care system to obtain more efficient and cost-effective patient care has resulted in many changes in personnel responsibilities. One of the major changes has been the shifting of blood specimen collection from phlebotomists based in the clinical laboratory to nurses and other allied health professionals that include certified nursing assistants, medical assistants, patient care technicians, respiratory therapists, radiographers, physician assistants, paramedics, and emergency medical technicians.

Consequently, many health-care personnel are now required to become proficient in a skill for which they have had little or no previous exposure. Like any other skill, collection of quality blood specimens begins by obtaining the didactic knowledge associated with the procedure. All procedures are written in accordance with the current standards of the Clinical and Laboratory Standards Institute (CLSI), formerly the National Committee for Clinical Laboratory Standards (NCCLS), and the current Occupational Safety & Health Administration (OSHA) guidelines and recommendations. The CLSI is an organization of representatives from the laboratory profession, industry, and government that develop and publish guidelines and standards for all areas of the laboratory, including blood collection. The responsibility of the CLSI is to ensure that all procedures are consistent with the current research and industry regulations. The didactic instruction is followed by performance of the skill with assistance and supervision. Adhering to proper technique and continued practice then becomes the key to acquiring proficiency. Regular competency assessments are required to evaluate the blood

1

collector's initial training and to ensure that the blood collector's performance continues to comply with the current standards.

Importance of Correct Specimen Collection and Handling

Laboratory testing of blood specimens is vital to the correct diagnosis, treatment, and monitoring of a patient's condition. Laboratory results constitute 70% of the objective information used by health-care providers to manage patient care and resolve patient health problems. The quality of a test result is only as good as the quality of the specimen analyzed. Therefore, reports from a suboptimal specimen can result in treatment that can be potentially harmful to the patient by overmedicating or undermedicating the patient with death being the worst patient outcome.

Laboratories are charged with the responsibility for specimen integrity by the Clinical Laboratory Improvement Amendments of 1988 (CLIA, 1988). These are federal regulations administered by the Centers for Medicare & Medicaid Services (CMS) to establish standards for reliable laboratory test results. In accordance to these standards, guidelines for specimen collection are published by the laboratory and should be available in all areas where patient samples are collected. Personnel collecting specimens should become familiar with these guidelines and refer to them or call the laboratory whenever they are unsure of a procedure.

Although the primary concern of personnel collecting blood specimens is understandably to obtain the specimen, failure to adhere to the collection procedure can compromise the integrity of a successfully collected specimen. Approximately 56% of laboratory error occurs during the preanalytic phase (processes that occur before testing of the sample) of laboratory testing. Influencing factors are the responsibilities of the blood collector and include:

- Monitoring of specimen ordering
- Correct patient identification
- Patient communication and safety
- Patient preparation
- Timing of collections
- Phlebotomy equipment
- Collection techniques
- Specimen labeling
- Specimen transportation to the laboratory
- Specimen processing

It is these ancillary factors that most frequently affect specimen integrity, resulting in specimen rejection by the laboratory. Therefore, emphasis in this course is placed on both technical and nontechnical factors that must be included in quality blood specimen collection.

Safety Precautions

In addition to the safety precautions specifically associated with blood collection, which are covered in this text, personnel must observe all standard precautions required in patient care. These include:

- Wearing appropriate personnel protective equipment (PPE)
- Observation of isolation practices
- Hand washing
- Using only needles with safety devices in the intended manner
- Disposal of entire assembled tube holder and needle after use

- Recording all accidental needlesticks and exposures as required by the OSHA mandated written exposure control plan. Post exposure prophylaxis (PEP) should be started when necessary.
- Disposal of contaminated materials in designated biohazard containers
- Decontamination of surfaces using an approved disinfectant, such as sodium hypochlorite (diluted 1:10, or 1:100 for routine decontamination) prepared weekly and stored in a plastic bottle

Blood collection poses a serious risk for exposure to blood-borne pathogens, such as human immunodeficiency virus (HIV), hepatitis B (HBV), and hepatitis C (HCV). HBV has been found to be stable in dried blood and blood products for up to 7 days. In laboratory studies, HIV has been detected up to 3 days after drying and can survive longer if frozen. Standard precautions must be strictly observed. Workstation countertops, equipment, and telephones must be disinfected daily or when visually contaminated. OSHA and the Centers for Disease Control and Prevention (CDC) mandate that gloves be worn at all times when collecting blood specimens. Gloves must be changed and hands washed between patients. The wearing of gloves does not eliminate the need for hand washing. Alcohol-based hand sanitizers are an accepted substitute for hand washing except when the hands are visibly contaminated or the blood collector has been in an isolation room in which the patient has been diagnosed with a *Clostridium difficile* infection. Gowns or lab coats are recommended apparel. Blood collectors should wear lab coats with knitted cuffs and pull the gloves over the cuffs to cover exposed skin. Blood sprays resulting from venipuncture or dermal puncture are likely to occur from the fingers to the elbows and from the collarbone to the waist.

Most blood-borne pathogen exposures associated with blood collection occur as a result of accidental puncture with a contaminated needle or lancet. A major significant exposure occurs when a deep puncture is caused by a needle that has been used to collect blood. Therefore, strict adherence to all safety precautions is essential.

Never recap needles and always discard them in puncture-resistant containers located close to the patient. The Needlestick Safety and Prevention Act of 2000 requires employers to provide sharps with engineered sharps injury protection features and to solicit employee input in selecting and reviewing these devices. A variety of safety devices for needle disposal and also a variety of protective needle sheaths are available (see Unit 2, Venipuncture Equipment). It is extremely important that personnel become totally familiar with the use of these safety devices. Many accidental punctures occur because personnel do not know how to properly use the available safety devices.

Blood collected using a syringe must be transferred to the appropriate evacuated tubes. This presents an additional safety risk, because in the past, the transfer procedure was to puncture the rubber stopper of the evacuated tube with the syringe needle and allow the blood to flow into the tube. This procedure is no longer recommended by the CLSI. The recommended safer technique is to use a blood transfer device (see Unit 2, Venipuncture Equipment). Removal of the rubber stopper, adding the blood from the syringe, and restoppering the tube is not recommended, because aerosols are produced and tubes are not as tightly stoppered for transport.

A well-stocked blood collection tray contains racks for tubes, needle disposal units, and additional supplies (see Unit 2). Therefore, a blood collection tray should be placed within close proximity to the patient whenever blood is being collected.

Personnel working in off-site facilities or physicians' offices may be required to perform initial specimen processing, such as centrifugation and separation of serum or plasma from blood cells. Centrifugation of uncapped tubes produces potentially harmful aerosols. Tubes must be carefully balanced in the centrifuge to prevent breakage, and the centrifuge lid must remain closed during operation to protect workers from exposure to blood and glass should a breakage occur. To prevent aerosol exposure when removing stoppers from evacuated tubes, first cover the stopper with gauze and then twist rather than "pop" off. Aerosols also are produced when specimens are poured rather than pipetted during transfer between tubes. A Plexiglas shield should be used when aliquoting specimens.

Specimens collected from home healthcare or nursing home patients and specimens being transported between physicians' offices and laboratories must be appropriately packaged for transport. Specimens for local transport should be placed in securely closed, leakproof primary containers (tubes and screw-top containers). The primary containers are enclosed in a secondary leakproof container with sufficient absorbent material present to separate the specimens and absorb the contents of the primary containers in case of leakage or breakage. Containers should be labeled as biohazardous. Specimens that are transported via a pneumatic tube system must be placed in a labeled biohazard plastic bag and correctly cushioned to avoid breakage of the tube or hemolysis of the blood.

Blood collection is safely performed only when personnel adhere to all recommended precautions.

SAFETY TIP

Needles used for blood collection have a greater potential for transmitting blood-borne pathogens than do needles used for other purposes. Report *all* needlesticks.

Types of Specimens

The laboratory refers to blood specimens primarily in terms of whole blood, plasma, and serum. A whole blood specimen contains erythrocytes, leukocytes, and platelets suspended in plasma and essentially represents blood as it circulates through the body. Tests related to blood cells, such as the complete blood count (CBC) and blood typing, are performed on whole blood.

The majority of laboratory tests are performed on the liquid portion of blood (plasma or serum), which contains substances, such as proteins, enzymes, organic and inorganic chemicals, and antibodies. Plasma is the liquid portion of blood that has not clotted; serum is the liquid portion remaining after clotting has occurred. Plasma is often defined as the liquid portion of blood that contains fibrinogen and other clotting factors, and serum as the liquid portion that does not contain fibrinogen and other clotting factors. Both serum and plasma are obtained by centrifugation of clotted and unclotted specimens, which separates the cellular elements from the liquid portion (**Fig. 1–1**).

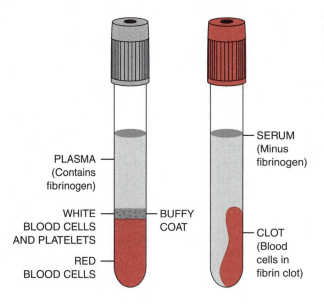

PLASMA
(Contains
fibrinogen)

WHITE
BLOOD CELLS
AND PLATELETS

RED
BLOOD CELLS

BUFFY
COAT

SERUM
(Minus
fibrinogen)

CLOT
(Blood
cells in
fibrin clot)

FIGURE 1–1. Differences between plasma and serum. *(Modified from Strasinger, SK, and Di Lorenzo, MA: Phlebotomy Workbook, ed. 2. FA Davis, Philadelphia, 2003, Figure 2–4, p. 21, with permission.)*

The presence or absence of anticoagulants in the tubes into which blood specimens are placed determines the type of specimen available for testing. Whole blood and plasma require an anticoagulant to prevent clot formation. Serum is obtained from tubes that do not contain an anticoagulant.

Collection tubes contain a variety of anticoagulants, the chemical content of which must be considered in conjunction with the laboratory test requested. As shown in **Figure 1–2,** anticoagulants prevent coagulation by two different mechanisms. The anticoagulants dipotassium (K_2) and tripotassium (K_3) ethylenediaminetetraacetic acid (EDTA), sodium citrate, and potassium oxalate bind calcium, which is required by the coagulation cascade. Heparin in the form of sodium, ammonium, or lithium heparin inhibits the formation of thrombin that is required to convert fibrinogen into a fibrin clot.

With the obvious exception of coagulation tests, many laboratory tests can be performed on either serum or plasma. However, the anticoagulant composition and method of action must be considered when tests are to be run on plasma. For example, an EDTA tube cannot be used when a plasma calcium level is requested, because the plasma calcium will be bound to the EDTA, resulting in falsely decreased values. Normal values of some analytes also differ between serum and plasma. Laboratory protocols for specimen collection specify the type of tube to be used. These protocols have been designed to ensure that the most representative test results are obtained, and they must be followed.

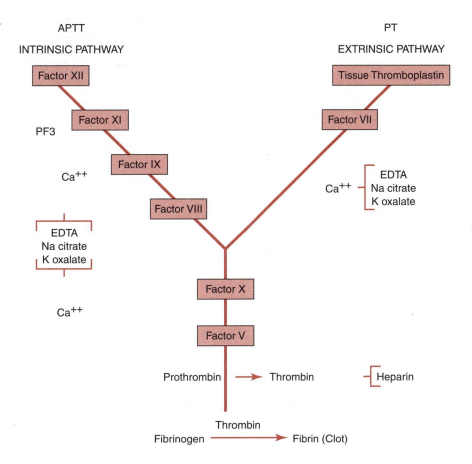

FIGURE 1–2. The role of anticoagulants in the coagulation cascade. (Ca = calcium; PF3 = platelet factor 3) *(Modified from Strasinger, SK, and Di Lorenzo, MA: Phlebotomy Workbook, ed. 2. FA Davis, Philadelphia, 2003, Figure 5–15, p. 93, with permission.)*

Normal serum and plasma appear clear and pale yellow. Variations in the normal appearance can indicate that certain test results may be adversely affected. Examples of abnormal appearance that are discussed in more detail later in the course include:

Hemolyzed – Pink to red color, indicating red blood cell destruction

Icteric – Dark yellow color, indicating the presence of increased bilirubin

Lipemic – Cloudy, milky appearance, indicating the presence of increased lipids

Venous blood is the specimen of choice for clinical laboratory testing, and most normal values are based on venous blood. However, tests also are performed on arterial and capillary specimens.

Arterial blood is the required specimen for arterial blood gas determinations. In the interest of patient safety, only specifically trained personnel must perform arterial punctures. Arterial blood also may be collected from central lines.

Capillary blood is a mixture of arterial and venous blood and is collected by dermal puncture. When properly collected, capillary blood is suitable for many laboratory tests, but normal values may differ from those of venous blood. Therefore, requisition forms should indicate whether the specimen is arterial or capillary blood.

> **TECHNICAL TIP**
>
> For anticoagulants to totally prevent clotting, specimens must be thoroughly mixed immediately following collection.

Quality Assurance

Laboratory quality assurance is designed to guarantee quality patient care by ensuring accurate and reliable test results in an appropriate and timely manner. As can be seen from this brief introduction, many factors related to blood collection can affect laboratory quality assurance. These factors are covered in detail in the following units. In addition, remember that laboratory personnel are available to answer questions and should be consulted whenever necessary.

Safety Situation Exercise

1. In the Obstetrics and Gynecology (OB/GYN) office, the physician ordered a urine pregnancy test, CBC, and a rubella titer on a young woman. The nurse drew the blood for the CBC and rubella titer and instructed the patient to collect a urine specimen in a prelabeled urine container. All specimens were placed together in a biohazard bag and sent by courier to the laboratory. When the specimen was received in the lab, half of the urine had spilled and leaked through the blood collection tube labels.

   a. Can the urine sample be used for the pregnancy test?

   _____

   b. What must be done to the blood collection tubes?

   _____
   _____
   _____

   c. How should these specimens have been transported?

   _____
   _____
   _____

d. What might the laboratory personnel do with the specimen?

_____

_____

_____

2. A patient in the infectious disease clinic needed blood drawn for an HBV test, HCV test, and an HIV test. It was the nurse's first day working in that clinic and the nurse was not familiar with the new blood collection equipment. The nurse easily performed the venipuncture and collected the blood but not being accustomed to the needle safety device, the nurse used a two-handed technique and fumbled to activate the safety device and accidentally stuck the left thumb with the contaminated needle.

a. What should the nurse do first?

_____

_____

_____

b. What tests are performed on the nurse?

_____

_____

c. If necessary, when should the nurse receive postexposure prophylaxis (PEP)?

_____

_____

_____

d. How could this accident have been avoided?

_____

_____

_____

REVIEW QUESTIONS

1. In addition to obtaining the blood specimen, the collector is responsible for:
   a. Correct patient identification
   b. The quality of the specimen
   c. Correct timing of the collection
   d. All of the above

2. Surfaces contaminated with blood must be cleaned using:
   a. Antibacterial soap
   b. Sodium hypochlorite
   c. Isopropyl alcohol
   d. Chlorhexidine

3. When transporting specimens to the laboratory from an off-site collection center, leakproof primary containers should be enclosed in:
   a. Sealed metal containers
   b. Leakproof secondary containers
   c. Absorbent material
   d. Both b and c

4. An anticoagulated, uncentrifuged blood specimen is called:
   a. Plasma
   b. Cellular blood
   c. Whole blood
   d. Serous blood

5. An evacuated tube containing EDTA cannot be used to collect a specimen for:
   a. A CBC
   b. Blood typing
   c. A calcium level
   d. Platelet counts

6. The liquid portion of blood collected in a nonanticoagulated tube is:
   a. Plasma
   b. Serum
   c. Whole blood
   d. Capillary blood

7. The liquid portion of blood collected in a heparinized tube is:
   a. Plasma
   b. Serum
   c. Whole blood
   d. Capillary blood

8. Which of the following pairings is incorrect?
   a. Hemolyzed: red
   b. Lipemic: cloudy
   c. Icteric: yellow
   d. None of the above

9. When an anticoagulated specimen is collected it must be immediately:
   a. Thoroughly mixed
   b. Placed on ice
   c. Taken to the laboratory
   d. Placed vertically in a test tube rack

10. Failure to become familiar with needle disposal equipment can result in:
    a. Hemolyzed specimens
    b. Failure to obtain the specimen
    c. A clotted anticoagulated specimen
    d. An accidental needlestick

Internet Help

http://www.cdc.gov/niosh/
    topics/bbp
http://www.clsi.org
http://www.fda.gov

http://www.osha.gov
http://www.osha.gov/SLTC/bloodbornepathogens

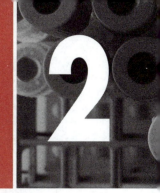

Venipuncture Equipment **2**

LEARNING OBJECTIVES

Upon completion of this unit, the reader will be able to:

- Discuss the use of a blood collection tray, transport carriers, and drawing stations.
- Differentiate between an evacuated tube system, syringe, and a winged blood collection set for the collection of blood by venipuncture.
- Differentiate among the various needle sizes as to length, gauge, and purpose.
- Discuss methods to safely dispose of contaminated needles.
- Identify the types of evacuated tubes by color code, and state the anticoagulants and additives present, the mechanism of action, any special characteristics, and the purpose of each.
- List the correct order of draw for the various types of blood collection tubes.
- Discuss the purpose and types of tourniquets.
- Name three substances used to cleanse the skin prior to venipuncture.
- Discuss the use of gloves, gauze, and bandages when performing venipuncture.
- Describe the quality control of venipuncture equipment.

Introduction

Considering the many types of blood specimens that may be required for laboratory testing and the risks to both patients and health-care personnel associated with blood collection, it is understandable that a considerable amount of equipment is required for the procedure.

This unit describes the various blood collection systems, collection tubes, order of draw, safety disposal systems, and other required supplies necessary for efficient blood collection.

Organization of Equipment

An important key to successful blood collection is making sure that all the required equipment is conveniently present in the collection area. Trays designed to organize and transport collection equipment are available from several manufacturers (**Fig. 2–1**). Maintaining a well-equipped blood collection tray that the blood collector carries into the patient's room (with the exception of isolation rooms) is the ideal way to prevent unnecessary errors during blood collection. Place the tray on a solid surface, such as a nightstand and not on the patient's bed, where it

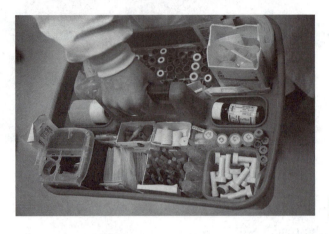

FIGURE 2–1. Blood collection tray.

can be knocked off. Trays should be emptied and disinfected on a weekly basis and more frequently if they become visibly soiled.

Mobile phlebotomy workstations with swivel-caster wheels have replaced the traditional phlebotomy tray in some institutions. With the increased amounts of required equipment necessary for safe phlebotomy, these versatile mobile workstations can be configured to accommodate phlebotomy trays, hazardous waste containers, sharps containers, and storage drawers and shelves. The cart is designed to be wheeled around the hospital and up to the patient's bedside to eliminate placing equipment or a phlebotomy tray on the patient's bed (**Fig. 2–2**).

In outpatient settings, use a blood drawing chair with an attached or adjacently placed stand to hold equipment (**Fig. 2–3**). Drawing chairs have an armrest that locks in place in front of the patient to properly position the arm and to provide arm support and protect the patient from falling out of the chair if he or she faints. A reclining chair or bed should be available for special procedures or for patients who feel faint or ill. Infant cradle pads are available for collection of blood from an infant (**Fig. 2–4**).

Venipuncture can be performed using an evacuated tube system, a syringe system, or a winged blood collection (butterfly) set. Each of these systems requires its own unique equipment, which is discussed in the following sections. Supplies that are common to all procedures also are discussed.

> **TECHNICAL TIP**
>
> A blood collector with well-organized equipment instills patient confidence.

Evacuated Tube System (ETS)

The evacuated tube system (**Fig. 2–5**) is the most frequently used method for performing venipuncture and is available from various manufacturers. Blood is collected directly into the evacuated tube, eliminating the need for transfer of specimens and minimizing the risk of biohazard exposure. The evacuated tube system consists of a double-pointed needle to puncture the stopper of the collection tube with one point and to puncture the patient's vein with the other point, a holder to hold the needle and collection tube, and color-coded evacuated tubes.

> **TECHNICAL TIP**
>
> It is recommended to not interchange evacuated tube system components from different manufacturers.

Needles

Sterile needles for venipuncture are disposable and used only once. Venipuncture needles include multisample needles, hypodermic needles, and winged blood collection (butterfly) needles. Multisample needles are packaged

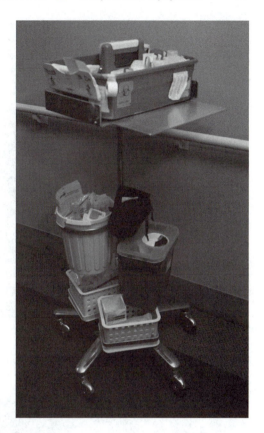

FIGURE 2–2. Mobile phlebotomy workstation.

in sterile, twist-apart sealed shields that are color-coded according to the size of the needle and must not be used if the seal is broken. Multisample needles used with an evacuated tube system are threaded in the middle and have a beveled point at each end. The front end is used to enter the vein, and the back end is used to penetrate the rubber stopper of an evacuated tube. A retractable rubber sheath covers the back end of the needle to prevent leakage of blood as tubes are changed or removed. Syringe hypodermic needles and winged blood collection set needles are packaged individually in sterile packets. All needles consist of a beveled point, shaft, lumen, and hub. **Figure 2–6** shows the difference between the hypodermic (syringe needle) and the multisample needle structures. Needles should be visually examined for structural defects, such as no beveled points or bent shafts, immediately before use. Defective needles should not be used. Needles should never be recapped once the shield is removed regardless of whether they have or have not been used.

Needle size varies by both length and gauge and is indicated by color-coded caps. The needle gauge refers to the diameter of the needle; the lower the number, the larger the needle. Needles range from 20- to 23-gauge for venipuncture; however, the standard needles used with evacuated tubes are 21- or 22-gauge with a 1-inch or 1.5-inch length. Although a 20-gauge needle will allow blood to flow more quickly, it is not recommended for routine blood collection. Many patients are on blood thinners and the use of a 20-gauge needle can result in postpuncture bleeding and hematomas because of the larger opening in the vein. Children and patients with small veins may require 23-gauge needles with a ¾ -inch length. Small volume pediatric evacuated tubes or partial

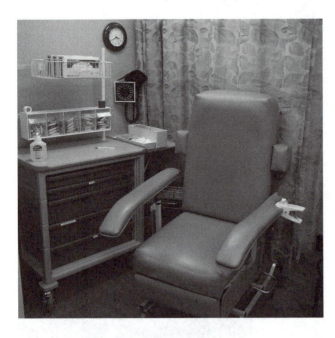

FIGURE 2–3. Phlebotomy drawing station, including a reclining chair.

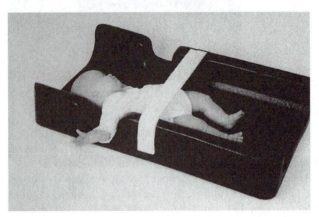

FIGURE 2–4. Infant cradle pad. *(Courtesy of Innovative Laboratory Acrylics, Inc., Brighton, MI.)*

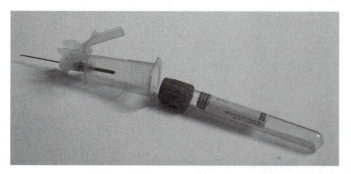

FIGURE 2–5. Evacuated tube system.

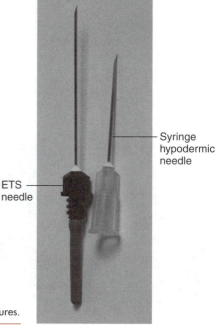

Syringe hypodermic needle

ETS needle

FIGURE 2–6. Needle structures.

draw tubes should be used with small-gauge needles because a small-diameter needle with a large evacuated tube can cause hemolysis as the blood is being pulled through the small lumen of the needle by the vacuum in the collection tubes. Using 25-gauge needles is not recommended because of the longer time the needle is in the vein and the increased frequency of hemolysis. The small lumen size of the 25-gauge needle causes the tube to fill more slowly and microclots may form. Needles used to collect units of blood for transfusion are the larger, 16-gauge needles.

Many needles are currently equipped with safety shields and blunting devices. The Occupational Safety and Health Administration (OSHA) has issued a directive mandating the evaluation and implementation of safety devices. State mandates also have been issued. Safety features include devices that blunt the needle, retract the needle after use, or shields that cover the needle after use. Safety shields covering the needles have been introduced with the SafetyGlide blood collection system (Becton, Dickinson, Franklin Lakes, NJ). The blood collector pushes the movable shield along the cannula with the thumb to enclose the needle tip after venipuncture (**Fig. 2–7**). The BD Vacutainer Eclipse blood collection needle utilizes a shield that the blood collector locks over the needle tip after completion of the venipuncture (**Fig. 2–8**). The Venipuncture Needle-Pro (Smiths Medical, St. Paul, MN) resheathes the needle by engaging the shield against a hard surface (**Fig. 2–9**).

Self-blunting needles (Punctur-Guard by Gaven Medical, Vernon, CT) are available to provide additional protection against needlestick injuries by making the needle blunt before removal from the patient. A hollow, blunt inner needle is contained inside the standard needle. Before removing the needle from the patient's vein, an additional push on the final tube in the holder advances the internal blunt cannula past the sharp tip of the outer needle. The blunt cannula is hollow, allowing blood to continue to flow into the tube (**Fig. 2–10**).

TECHNICAL TIP

Many health-care workers feel that they have better control using a 1-inch needle.

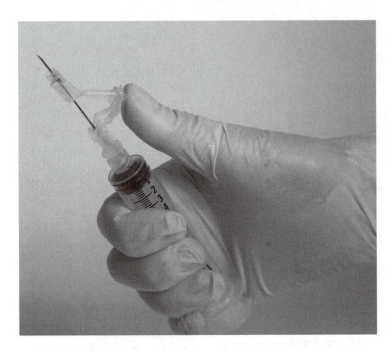

FIGURE 2–7. SafetyGlide blood collection assembly.

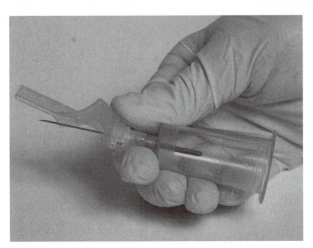

FIGURE 2–8. Eclipse blood collection needle.

Holders

Needle holders used with evacuated collection systems are designed to accommodate different sizes of collection tubes. Holders are made of clear, rigid plastic and are available with or without safety features. Various holders are shown in **Figure 2–11.**

The back end of the evacuated tube system needle screws securely into the holder. The first tube is partially advanced onto the stopper-puncturing needle up to a designated mark on the holder. Pushing the tube beyond this point will break the tube's vacuum, making the tube unusable. The tube is fully advanced onto the end of the holder when the needle is in the vein.

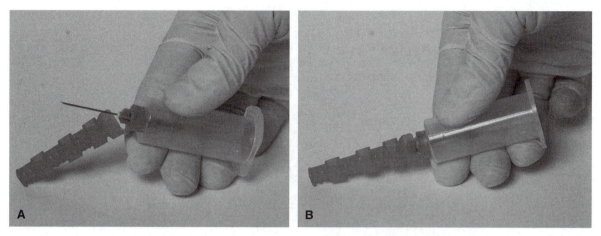

FIGURE 2–9. Venipuncture Needle-Pro. *A,* Activating shield on a hard surface. *B,* Shield fully engaged.

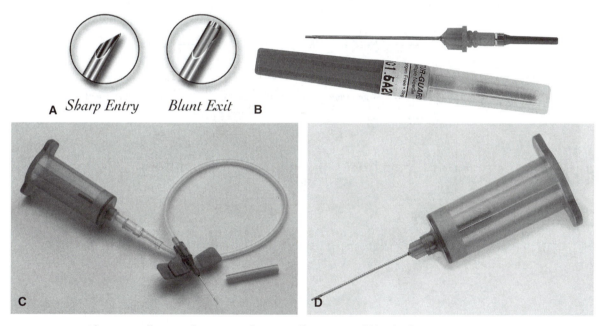

FIGURE 2–10. Blunting needle principle. *A,* Principle. *B,* Needle. *C,* Winged blood collection set. *D,* Multisample needle attached to holder. *(Courtesy of Gaven Medical, Vernon, CT.)*

Blood will flow into the tube once the needle penetrates the stopper. The flared ends of the holder aid the blood collector during the changing of tubes in multiple-draw situations **(Fig. 2–12)**. Tubes are removed with a slight twist to help disengage them from the needle.

In June 2002, OSHA issued a revision to the Bloodborne Pathogens Standard compliance directive. In the revised directive, the agency requires that all blood holders with needles

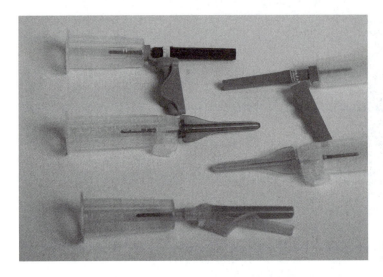

FIGURE 2–11. Various types of tube holders.

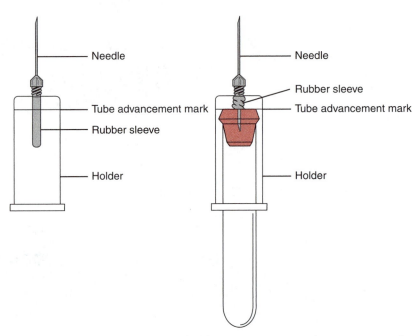

FIGURE 2–12. Needle holder. *(Modified from Strasinger, SK, and Di Lorenzo, MS: The Phlebotomy Workbook, edition 2, FA Davis, Philadelphia, 2003, Figure 12-5, p. 177, with permission.)*

attached be immediately discarded into a sharps container after the device's safety feature is activated. Rationale for the new directive is based on the exposure of workers to the unprotected stopper-puncturing end of evacuated tube needles, the increased needle manipulation required to remove it from the holder, and the possible worker exposure from the use of contaminated holders.

TECHNICAL TIP

Loss of tube vacuum is a primary cause of failure to obtain blood. The venipuncture can be performed prior to placing the tube on the needle. Practice both methods and choose the one with which you are most comfortable.

SAFETY TIP

If the evacuated tube needle does not have a safety device, the tube holder must have a safety shield.

SAFETY TIP

To prevent accidental punctures from contaminated needles, become thoroughly familiar with the operation of your needle safety system before performing blood collection.

Several safety holders are available that include a protective shield that covers the needle after use or automatically retracts the needle into the holder after venipuncture (**Fig. 2–13**). Venipuncture Needle-Pro (Smiths Medical, St. Paul, MN) utilizes a plastic shield attached by a hinge to the end of the evacuated tube holder. The shield hangs free during the venipuncture and when engaged against a hard surface, the needle is encapsulated by the shield. The entire device is discarded in the sharps container. The ProGuard II safety needle holder (Covidien, Mansfield, MA) uses a one-handed method to retract the needle into the holder and a cover for the end that is open to the stopper-puncturing needle. The Vanish Point tube holder (Retractable Technologies, Little Elm, TX) automatically retracts the needle by securely closing the end cap while the needle is still in the patient's vein (**Fig. 2–14**).

Needle Disposal Systems

Needles must always be placed in rigid, puncture-resistant, leakproof disposable containers labeled BIOHAZARD that are easily sealed when full. Syringes with the needles attached, winged blood collection sets, and holders with needles attached are disposed of directly into puncture-resistant containers (**Fig. 2–15**).

Collection Tubes

The collection tubes used with the evacuated system (**Fig. 2–16**) are available in a variety of sizes and volumes ranging from 1.8 to 15 mL. The tubes are labeled with the type of anticoagulant or additive, the draw volume, and the expiration date. Evacuated tubes have color-coded rubber stoppers or plastic shields covering the rubber stoppers (Becton Dickinson Hemogard Vacutainer System, Franklin Lakes, NJ) to indicate the presence or absence of an additive or anticoagulant in the tube. The color-coding is generally universal; however, it may vary slightly by manufacturer, and describes the type of tube to use for sample collection, for example, "draw one red stopper and one light blue stopper tube." This reference to tube color is found on most computer-generated requisition forms. Each laboratory department has specific specimen requirements for the analysis of particular blood constituents.

FIGURE 2–13. Venipuncture Needle-Pro, Vanish-Point, BD holders.

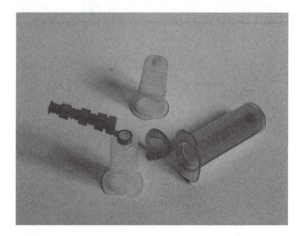

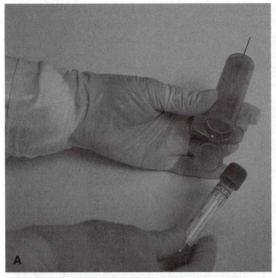

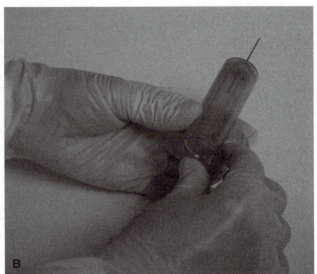

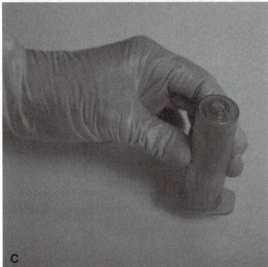

FIGURE 2–14. Vanish Point tube holder. *A,* Tube removed from holder. *B,* Activating shield. *C,* Needle retracted and holder sealed.

As shown in **Figure 2–17,** evacuated tubes have thick rubber stoppers with a thinner central area to allow puncture by the needle. Tubes may have a color-coded plastic safety shield covering the stopper to provide additional protection against blood splatter (BD Hemogard Vacutainer System) when stoppers are removed. Tubes are designed to be placed on the laboratory instrument and can be bar coded for identification and sampled directly by means of an instrument probe that pierces the stopper.

Evacuated tubes fill automatically because a premeasured vacuum is present in the tube. This causes some tubes to fill almost to the top, whereas other tubes only partially fill. Partial fill tubes have translucent colored Hemogard closures in the same color as regular fill tubes to distinguish them. The draw volume is written on the tube label. Tubes are sterile and silicone coated to prevent cells from adhering to the wall of the tube, thereby decreasing hemolysis.

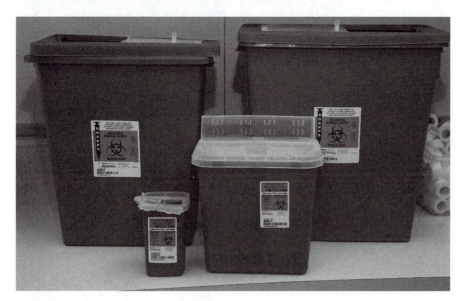

FIGURE 2–15. Sharps disposal containers.

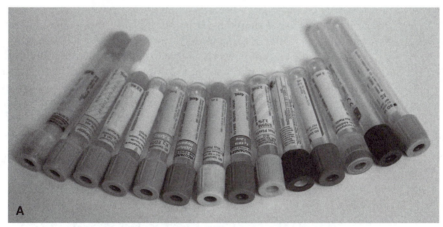

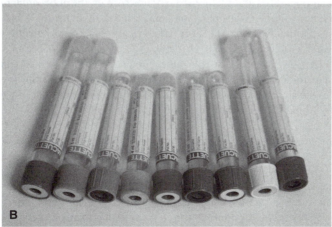

FIGURE 2–16. Evacuated tubes. *A,* BD Vacutainer tubes *(Becton Dickinson, Franklin Lakes, NJ). B,* Vacuette evacuated tubes *(Greiner Bio-One, Monroe, NC).*

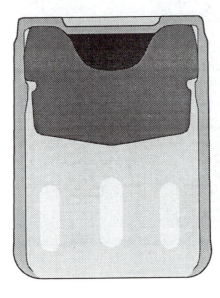

FIGURE 2–17. Cut-away view of a vacuum tube stopper (Hemogard closure). *(Adapted from product literature, Becton Dickinson, Franklin Lakes, NJ.)*

Tests requiring whole blood or plasma are collected in tubes containing an anticoagulant. Different types of anticoagulants are required for specific tests. All tubes containing an anticoagulant must be gently inverted three to eight times immediately after collection to mix the contents and to avoid microclot formation. Tubes containing an anticoagulant must be completely filled to the designated volume draw. If the blood-to-anticoagulant ratio is incorrect, test results may be erroneous. Partial collection tubes should be used when a short draw is anticipated. Additives present in evacuated tubes are used as preservatives and clot activators. Tubes containing additives also must be gently mixed to ensure effectiveness. Blood collected in a tube containing an anticoagulant or additive cannot be transferred into a tube containing a different anticoagulant or additive.

> **TECHNICAL TIP**
>
> Shaking an anticoagulated tube rather than gently inverting the tube may cause hemolysis and the specimen will be rejected.

COLOR-CODING OF TUBES

Lavender stopper tubes and Hemogard closures contain the anticoagulant EDTA in the form of liquid tripotassium (K_3EDTA) (glass) or spray-coated dipotassium ethylenediaminetetraacetic acid (K_2EDTA) (plastic). Coagulation is prevented by the binding of calcium in the specimen to sites on the large EDTA molecule, thereby preventing the participation of the calcium in the coagulation cascade (see Fig. 1–2). Lavender stopper tubes should be gently inverted eight times for adequate mixing. For hematology procedures that require whole blood, such as the complete blood count (CBC), K_2EDTA is the anticoagulant of choice because it maintains cellular integrity better than other anticoagulants, inhibits platelet clumping, and does not interfere with routine staining procedures. In an underfilled EDTA tube, the excess anticoagulant may shrink red blood cells and affect hematology tests. However, the tubes can be submitted to the laboratory for evaluation if necessary. The Clinical and Laboratory Standards Institute (CLSI) recommends K_2EDTA for hematology tests because liquid K_3EDTA dilutes the specimen and results in lower results. K_2EDTA tubes may be used for immunohematology testing and blood donor screening. Lavender stopper tubes cannot be used for coagulation studies because EDTA interferes with factor V and the thrombin-fibrinogen reaction.

Pink stopper tubes and Hemogard closures also contain a spray-coated K_2EDTA anticoagulant and are used specifically for blood bank in some facilities. Using a designated tube for a blood bank is believed to help prevent testing of specimens from the wrong patient. The tubes are designed with special labels for patient information required by the American Association of Blood Banks (AABB). Tubes should be inverted eight times.

White Hemogard closure tubes containing a spray-coated K_2EDTA anticoagulant and a separation gel are called plasma preparation tubes (PPTs). This differentiates them from plasma separator tubes that contain heparin as the anticoagulant. White Hemogard closure tubes are primarily used for molecular diagnostics test methods but can be used for myocardial infarction (MI) panels and ammonia levels, depending on the test methodology and instrumentation. Greiner Bio-One K_2EDTA tubes with gel have a lavender stopper with a yellow top. Tubes should be inverted eight times.

> **TECHNICAL TIP**
>
> Overmixing a light blue stopper tube can activate platelets and produce erroneous coagulation test results.

> **TECHNICAL TIP**
>
> The laboratory always rejects incompletely filled light blue stopper tubes.

> **TECHNICAL TIP**
>
> Underfilled sodium citrate tubes will have an incorrect anticoagulant to blood ratio, which can cause a falsely lengthened APTT result.

Light blue stopper tubes and Hemogard closures contain the anticoagulant sodium citrate, which also prevents coagulation by binding calcium. Centrifugation of the anticoagulated light blue stopper tubes provides the plasma used for coagulation tests. Sodium citrate is the required anticoagulant for coagulation studies because it preserves the labile coagulation factors. CTAD light blue stopper tubes contain citrate, theophylline, adenosine, and dipyridamole and are used for selected platelet function assays. Greiner Bio-One CTAD tubes have blue stoppers with yellow tops. Tubes should be gently inverted three to four times.

The ratio of blood to liquid sodium citrate is critical and should be 9:1 (example: 4.5 mL blood and 0.5 mL sodium citrate). This tube requires a full draw to prevent dilution of coagulation factors. When drawing coagulation tests on patients with polycythemia or hematocrit readings more than 55 percent, the amount of anticoagulant must be decreased to maintain the 9:1 ratio, because the lower volume of plasma in these patients will be diluted by the standard volume of sodium citrate. Likewise, the amount of anticoagulant must be increased for severely anemic patients because of the larger amount of plasma. The laboratory should be consulted to provide tubes with the appropriate amount of anticoagulant.

A special dark blue stopper tube containing thrombin and a soybean trypsin inhibitor must be used when drawing blood for determinations of certain fibrin degradation products.

Black stopper tubes containing sodium citrate are used for Westergren erythrocyte sedimentation rates (ESR). They differ from light blue stopper tubes in that they provide a ratio of blood to liquid anticoagulant of 4:1. Specially designed tubes for Westergren erythrocyte sedimentation rates are available.

Green stopper tubes and Hemogard closures contain the anticoagulant heparin combined with sodium, lithium, or ammonium ion. Heparin prevents clotting by inhibiting thrombin in the coagulation cascade (**see Fig. 1–2**). Tubes should be mixed eight times by gentle inversion to mix the specimen and to prevent hemolysis. Green stopper tubes are used for chemistry tests performed on whole blood or plasma. Interference by sodium and lithium heparin with their corresponding chemical tests and by ammonium heparin in blood urea nitrogen (BUN) determinations must be avoided. Green stopper tubes are not used for hematology because heparin interferes with the Wright stained blood smear used for differentials.

Light green Hemogard closure tubes and **green/black** stopper tubes contain lithium heparin and a separation gel and are called plasma separator tubes (PST). PST tubes are used for plasma determinations in chemistry. They are well suited for potassium determinations because heparin prevents the release of potassium by platelets during clotting and the gel prevents contamination of the plasma by red blood cell potassium. Mix by gentle inversion eight times. With the Greiner Bio-One blood collection tubes, the heparinized gel tubes have green plastic stoppers with yellow tops.

Gray stopper tubes and Hemogard closures are available with a variety of additives and antico-agulants for the primary purpose of preserving glucose. All gray stopper tubes contain a glucose preservative (antiglycolytic agent), sodium fluoride. Sodium fluoride maintains glucose for 3 days. Sodium fluoride is not an anticoagulant; therefore, if plasma is needed for analysis, anticoagulant must also be present. In gray stopper tubes, the anticoagulant is potassium oxalate or Na_2 EDTA that prevent clotting by binding calcium. When monitoring patient glucose levels, tubes for the collection of plasma and serum should not be interchanged. Gray stopper tubes should not be used for other chemical analyses because sodium fluoride interferes with some enzyme analyses that include creatine kinase (CK), alanine aminotransferase (ALT), aspartate aminotransferase (AST), or alkaline phosphatase (ALP). Gray stopper tubes are not used in hematology because potassium oxalate distorts cellular morphology.

Blood alcohol levels are drawn in gray stopper tubes containing sodium fluoride because microbial growth, which could produce alcohol as a metabolic end product, is inhibited. Tubes with or without potassium oxalate can be used, depending on the need for plasma or serum in the test procedure. Tubes are mixed eight times by gentle inversion.

Royal blue stopper tubes and Hemogard closures are used for trace elements, toxicology, and nutrient determinations. Because many of the elements analyzed in these studies are significant at very low levels, the tubes must be chemically clean to prevent contamination from the stopper material that could falsely elevate test results. The rubber stoppers are specially formulated to contain the lowest possible levels of metal or other contaminants. Royal blue stopper tubes are available with a clot activator, or with sodium heparin, or with K_2EDTA to conform to a variety of testing requirements. Tube labels are color-coded to indicate the type of additive or anticoagulant in the tube. Invert tubes with anticoagulants eight times and tubes with a clot activator five times to mix.

Tan Hemogard closure tubes are available for lead determinations. They are certified to contain less than 0.01 mcg/mL (ppm) lead. The tubes contain K_2EDTA anticoagulant and must be inverted eight times for proper mixing.

Yellow stopper tubes are available for two different purposes and contain different additives. Yellow stoppers are found on tubes containing the red blood cell preservative acid citrate dextrose (ACD). Specimens collected in these tubes are used for blood bank special cellular studies, human leukocyte antigen (HLA) phenotyping, and DNA and paternity testing. The acid citrate prevents clotting by binding calcium and the dextrose preserves the red blood cells. The tubes should be inverted eight times.

Sterile **yellow** stopper tubes containing the anticoagulant sodium polyanethol sulfonate (SPS) are used to collect specimens to be cultured for the presence of microorganisms. SPS aids in the recovery of microorganisms by inhibiting the actions of complement, phagocytes, and certain antibiotics. SPS binds calcium to prevent coagulation and the tube must be inverted eight times.

Yellow/gray rubber stoppers and **orange Hemogard closures** are found on tubes containing the clot activator thrombin. The addition of thrombin to the tube results in faster clot formation, usually within 5 minutes. Tubes containing thrombin are used for stat serum chemistry determinations and on samples from patients receiving anticoagulant therapy. Tubes should be inverted eight times.

Red/gray rubber stoppers and **gold Hemogard closures** are found on tubes containing a clot activator and a polymer separation gel. They are referred to as serum separator tubes (SST). The tubes contain silica that increases platelet activation, thereby shortening the time required for clot formation. Tubes should be inverted five times to expose the blood to the clot activator. A barrier polymer gel that undergoes a temporary change in viscosity during centrifugation is located at the bottom of the tube. As shown in **Figure 2–18,** when the tube is centrifuged, the gel forms a barrier between the cells and serum to prevent contamination of the serum with cellular materials.

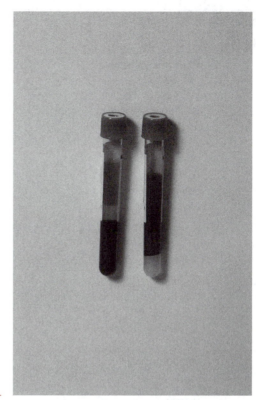

FIGURE 2–18. Serum separator tubes before and after collection and centrifugation.

To produce a solid separation barrier, specimens must be allowed to clot completely before centrifuging. Blood clotting time is usually 30 minutes and specimens should be centrifuged as soon as clot formation is complete. Serum separator tubes are used for most chemistry tests. They prevent contamination of the serum by cellular chemicals and products of cellular metabolism. They are not suitable for blood bank and certain immunology/serology tests. With the Greiner Bio-One blood collection tubes, the serum gel tubes have red plastic stoppers with yellow tops.

Red stopper plastic tubes and Hemogard closures also are available and these tubes contain silica as a clot activator. They are used for serum chemistry tests, serology tests, and in blood banks, where both serum and red blood cells may be used. The tubes are inverted five times to initiate the clotting process.

Red stopper glass tubes and Hemogard closures are often referred to as clot or plain tubes because they contain no anticoagulants or additives. Blood collected in red stopper glass tubes clots by the normal coagulation process in about 60 minutes. Centrifugation of the specimen then yields serum as the liquid portion. Red stopper tubes are used for the same purpose as the red plastic tubes. There is no need to invert glass red stopper tubes.

Red/light gray rubber stopper and clear Hemogard closures are plain tubes because they contain no anticoagulants, additives, or gel. They are used as a discard tube or secondary specimen collection tube. No inverting of the tube is required.

Evacuated tubes are summarized in **Table 2–1.** Appendix B lists laboratory tests and the required types of anticoagulants and volume of blood required.

TECHNICAL TIP

Centrifugation of incompletely clotted SST tubes can produce a nonintact gel barrier and possible cellular contamination of the serum.

TABLE 2–1. Summary of Evacuated Tubes

STOPPER COLOR	ANTICOAGULANT/ADDITIVE	SPECIMEN TYPE	LABORATORY USE
Lavender	Ethylenediaminetetraacetic acid (EDTA)	Whole blood/plasma	Hematology
Pink	EDTA	Whole blood/plasma	Blood bank
White	EDTA and gel	Plasma	Molecular diagnostics
Light blue	Sodium citrate	Plasma	Coagulation
Red/gray, gold	Clot activator and gel	Serum	Chemistry
Green	Ammonium heparin	Whole blood/plasma	Chemistry
	Lithium heparin	Whole blood/plasma	
	Sodium heparin	Whole blood/plasma	
Light green, green/black	Lithium heparin and gel	Plasma	Chemistry
Red (glass)	None	Serum	Blood bank, chemistry, serology
Red (plastic)	Clot activator	Serum	Chemistry, serology
Yellow/gray, orange	Thrombin	Serum	Chemistry
Gray	Potassium oxalate/sodium fluoride	Plasma	Chemistry glucose tests
	Sodium fluoride	Serum	
	Sodium fluoride/Na$_2$EDTA	Plasma	
Tan	K$_2$EDTA	Plasma	Chemistry lead tests
Royal blue	Sodium heparin	Plasma	Chemistry trace elements, toxicology, and nutrient analyses
	K$_2$EDTA	Plasma	
	Clot activator	Serum	
Yellow	Sodium polyanethol sulfonate (SPS)	Whole blood	Microbiology blood cultures
	Acid citrate dextrose (ACD)	Whole blood	Blood bank
Black	Sodium citrate	Whole blood	Hematology sedimentation rates
Red/light gray/clear	None		Discard tube

Order of Draw

Often several tests are ordered on patients, and blood must be collected in different tubes. The order in which tubes are drawn is one of the most important considerations when collecting blood specimens, as this can affect some test results. Tubes must be collected in a specific order to prevent invalid test results caused by contamination of the specimen by microorganisms, tissue thromboplastin, or carryover of additives or anticoagulants between tubes.

For example, the release of tissue thromboplastin from the skin as it is punctured can result in its presence in the first tube collected, and this could interfere with coagulation tests. Therefore, a light blue stopper tube should not be drawn first. If only a coagulation test is ordered, it is recommended that a few milliliters of blood be drawn into another light blue stopper tube or a clear "discard" tube and discarded. Recent studies suggest that the discard tube may no longer be necessary for routine coagulation tests (activated partial thromboplastin time

[APTT] and prothrombin time [PT]) unless the draw is difficult or when using a winged blood collection set, but it is still required for special coagulation tests. It is important that the blood collector follow the blood collection protocol of the facility.

Transfer of anticoagulants when changing tubes as a result of possible contamination of the stopper-puncturing needle must be avoided. Blood remaining on the needle after puncturing a tube can be transferred to the next tube. This is why the discard tube is drawn before the coagulation tube and why tubes containing anticoagulants are drawn after the light blue stopper tube. When one considers the mechanisms of anticoagulation and the chemical composition of the various anticoagulants, it can be understood that the results of several frequently requested tests could be compromised by contamination. For example, contamination of a green, red, or gold stopper tube designated for sodium, potassium, and calcium determinations with EDTA, sodium citrate, or potassium oxalate would falsely decrease the calcium and elevate the sodium or potassium results. Holding blood collection tubes in a downward position to ensure that the tubes fill from the bottom up helps avoid the transfer of anticoagulants from tube to tube. **Table 2–2** lists tests potentially affected by anticoagulant or additive contamination.

When sterile specimens, such as blood cultures, are to be collected, they must be considered in the order of draw. Such specimens are always drawn first in a sterile bottle or tube to prevent microbial contamination of the stopper puncturing needle from the unsterile stoppers of tubes used for the collection of other tests.

The CLSI recommends the following order of draw for both evacuated tube system and when filling tubes from a syringe:

- Sterile specimens (yellow, blood culture bottles)
- Light blue stopper tubes (sodium citrate)
- Serum tubes: Red/gray SST, gold SST, red plastic stopper tubes (clot activator), and red glass tubes
- Green stopper tubes and light green PST tubes (heparin)
- Lavender, pink, white (PPT), tan, and royal blue stopper tubes (EDTA)
- Gray stopper tubes (oxalate, fluoride)
- Yellow/gray or orange stopper tubes (thrombin clot activator)

Syringes

Syringes may be preferred over an evacuated tube system when drawing blood from patients with small or fragile veins. The advantage of this system is that the amount of suction pressure on the vein can be controlled by slowly pulling back the syringe plunger.

Syringes consist of a barrel graduated in milliliters (mL) or cubic centimeters (cc) and a plunger that fits tightly within the barrel creating a vacuum when retracted (**Fig. 2–19**). Syringes used for venipuncture range from 2 to 10 mL, and the blood collector should use a size that corresponds to the amount of blood needed. Needles are attached to a plastic hub designed to fit on the barrel of the syringe. The technique for use of syringes is discussed in Unit 4.

Syringes that provide a protective sheath to cover the needle before disposal are available. Examples of safety devices for syringe needles include the Hypodermic Needle-Pro (Smiths Medical, St. Paul, MN), the BD Hypodermic Eclipse needle, and the BD SafetyGlide hypodermic needle (Becton, Dickinson, Franklin Lakes, NJ) and are shown in **Figure 2–20.**

Blood drawn in a syringe must be immediately transferred to appropriate evacuated tubes to prevent the formation of clots. In the past, blood was transferred by puncturing the rubber stopper with the syringe needle and allowing the blood to be drawn, but not forced, into the tube. This is now considered unsafe according to the CLSI standards. Blood transfer devices provide a safer means for blood transfer when collecting blood with a syringe. It is an evacuated tube holder with

TABLE 2–2. Tests Affected by Anticoagulant/Additive Contamination

ANTICOAGULANT/ADDITIVE	POSSIBLE COMPROMISED TEST
Clot activator (silica)	Partial thromboplastin time
	Prothrombin time
EDTA	Activated partial thromboplastin time
	Alkaline phosphatase
	Calcium
	Creatine kinase
	Iron
	Potassium
	Prothrombin time
	Sodium
Heparin	Activated clotting time
	Acid phosphatase
	Activated partial thromboplastin time
	Ammonia (ammonium heparin)
	Blood urea nitrogen (ammonium heparin)
	Prothrombin time
	Sodium (sodium heparin)
	Lithium (lithium heparin)
Potassium oxalate	Acid phosphatase
	Activated partial thromboplastin time
	Alkaline phosphatase
	Amylase
	Calcium
	Lactate dehydrogenase
	Potassium
	Prothrombin time
	Red cell morphology
Sodium citrate	Alkaline phosphatase
	Calcium
	Phosphorus
Sodium fluoride	Blood urea nitrogen
	Sodium

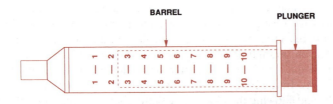

BARREL   PLUNGER

FIGURE 2–19. Diagram of a syringe. (Modified from Strasinger, SK, and Di Lorenzo, MS: Phlebotomy Workbook, ed. 2. FA Davis, Philadelphia, 2003, Figure 5-17, p. 98, with permission.)

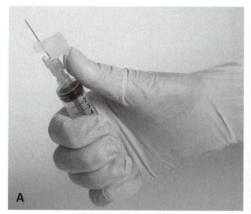

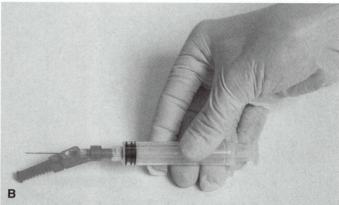

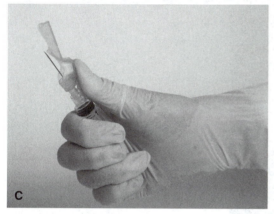

FIGURE 2–20. Syringe safety devices. *A,* Syringe with BD SafetyGlide needle attached. *B,* Syringe with Smiths Medical Hypodermic Needle-Pro. *C,* BD Eclipse hypodermic needle attached to a syringe.

a rubber-sheathed needle inside. After blood collection, the syringe tip is inserted into the hub of the device and evacuated tubes are filled by pushing them onto the rubber-sheathed needle in the holder as in an evacuated tube system (**Fig. 2–21**). The entire syringe/holder assembly is discarded in the sharps container after use. When tubes are filled from a syringe, CLSI recommends that tubes be filled in the same order as recommended for the order of draw previously listed. Some institutions, however, feel that because the portion of blood possibly contaminated by tissue thromboplastin is the first portion to enter the syringe, it is the last to be expelled. At these institutions, the order of transfer should be:

- Sterile specimens
- Light blue stopper tubes
- Other anticoagulants and additives
- Lavender stopper tube
- Green stopper tube
- Gray stopper tube
- Red, SST, or orange stopper tubes

Institutional policy should be followed.

TECHNICAL TIP

Let the vacuum in the evacuated tube draw the appropriate amount of blood into the tube. Discard any extra blood left in the syringe; do not force it into the tube.

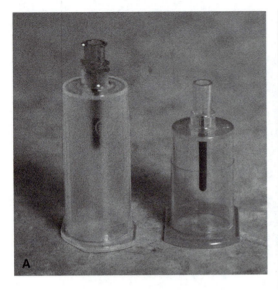

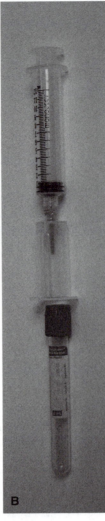

FIGURE 2–21. *A,* BD Transfer device *(Becton, Dickinson, Franklin Lakes, NJ)* and Saf-T Holder device *(Smiths Medical, St. Paul, MN). B,* Transfer device with tube.

Winged Blood Collection Sets

Winged blood collection sets, or butterflies as they are routinely called, are used for:

- The infusion of IV fluids
- Performing venipuncture from very small veins
- Obtaining specimens from children and the elderly

Winged blood collection needles used for phlebotomy are usually 23-gauge with lengths of ½ to ¾ inch. Plastic attachments to the needle, which resemble butterfly wings, are used for holding the needle during insertion and to secure the apparatus during IV therapy. They also provide the ability to lower the needle insertion angle when working with very small veins. To

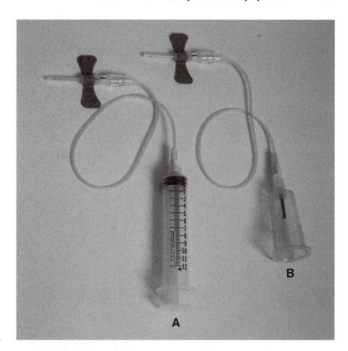

FIGURE 2–22. Winged blood collection sets. *A,* Attached to a syringe. *B,* Attached to an evacuated tube holder.

accommodate the dual purpose of venipuncture and infusion, the needle is attached to flexible plastic tubing that can be attached to an IV setup, syringe, or specially designed evacuated tube adapters (**Fig. 2–22**).

There are several winged blood collection needle sets with safety devices built into the system (**Fig. 2–23**). The Vacutainer Safety-Lok (Becton, Dickinson) uses a retractable safety enclosure that covers the needle once it has been withdrawn. After use, the needle is completely retracted into the protective shield and locked in place by pushing the yellow shield forward. The BD Vacutainer Push Button Collection set uses in-vein activation of the needle. The needle is automatically retracted into the device when the blood collector pushes the activation button with the index finger while the needle is still in the vein. Another widely used needle set is the Monoject Angel Wing blood collection set (Kendall, Mansfield, MA). When the needle is withdrawn, a stainless steel safety shield is activated and locks in place to cover the needle. The Puncture Guard winged infusion set (Gaven Medical, Vernon, CT) produces a safety device that blunts the needle before withdrawal from the vein (**Fig. 2–24**).

The technique for the use of winged blood collection sets is covered in Unit 4.

Combination Systems

The S-Monovette Blood Collection System (Sarstedt, Inc., Newton, NC) is an enclosed multisampling blood collection system that includes the blood collection tube and collection device. Blood is collected using either an aspiration or vacuum principle of collection with multisampling needles with preassembled holders, needle protection devices, and a safety winged blood collection set (**Fig. 2–25**).

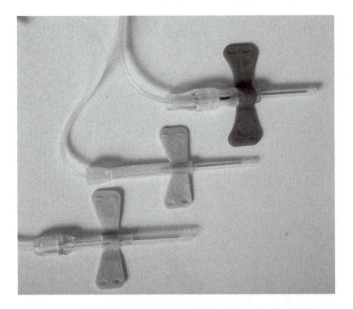

FIGURE 2-23. Examples of winged blood collection sets.

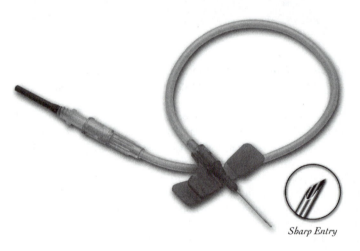

Sharp Entry   *Blunt Exit*

FIGURE 2-24. Puncture Guard Winged Blood Collection Set. *(Gaven Medical, Vernon, CT.)*

Tourniquets

Tourniquets are used during venipuncture to make it easier to locate a patient's veins. They do this by impeding venous, but not arterial, blood flow in the area just below the tourniquet application site. The distended vein then becomes more visible and palpable.

The most frequently used tourniquets are flat latex or vinyl strips (**Fig. 2-26**). They are inexpensive and may be disposed of between patients or reused if disinfected. Tourniquets with Velcro and buckle closures are easier to apply but are more difficult to decontaminate. The advantage of a buckle closure tourniquet is that it stays on the patient's arm and can be retightened if necessary. Rubber tubing may be used for pediatric patients. Flat nonlatex strips are available for persons allergic to latex. Rolls of disposable nonlatex strips are available for one-time use.

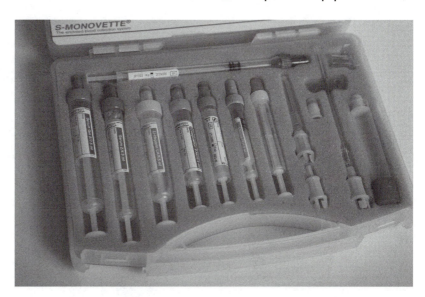

FIGURE 2–25. S-Monovette Blood Collection System. *(Sarstedt, Inc., Newton, NC.)*

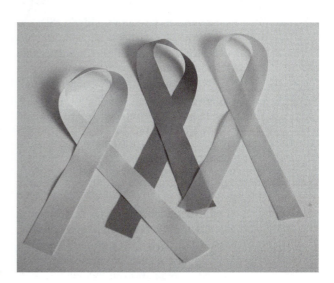

FIGURE 2–26. Various types of tourniquets.

Blood pressure cuffs can be used as tourniquets. The cuff should be inflated to a pressure of 40 mm Hg to allow blood to flow into but not out of the affected veins. The application of tourniquets and the effects on blood tests are discussed in Units 3 and 4.

Vein-Locating Devices

Portable devices are available to locate veins that are not easily visible. They are particularly advantageous for the neonatal, pediatric, and frail adult patient populations to avoid multiple needlestick attempts for blood collection and for IV insertion. The Venoscope II (**Fig. 2–27**) and Neonatal Transilluminator (Venoscope, LLC, Lafayette, LA) and the Transillumination Vein Locator (VL-U) (Promedic, McCordsville, IN) use a high-intensity LED light that shines through the patient's

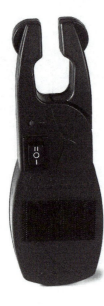

FIGURE 2–27. Venoscope II trans-illuminator device. *(Courtesy of Venoscope, LLC, Lafayette, LA.)*

subcutaneous tissue to highlight the veins that absorb the light rather than reflecting it. The vein stands out as a dark line allowing the blood collector to note the direction of the vein. The blood collector then marks the vein for needle insertion. The Vena-Vue (Biosynergy, Elk Grove Village, IL) uses liquid crystal thermography to locate veins. The device is placed on the skin like a bandage to cool the skin. Heat-emitting veins appear that the blood collector can feel and mark for reassurance. The Vein Entry Indicator Device (VEID) (Vascular Technologies, Ness-Ziona, Israel) uses a sensor technology to indicate correct insertion of a catheter needle in a vein. The device emits a continuous beeping signal indicating a change of pressure when the needle penetrates a blood vessel. The beeping signal stops when the needle exits the vein.

Gloves

OSHA mandates that gloves must be worn when collecting blood and must be changed after each patient. Under routine circumstances, gloves do not need to be sterile. To provide maximal manual dexterity, they should fit securely.

Gloves are available in several varieties, including powdered and powder-free and latex and nonlatex. Nonlatex can include nitrile, neoprene, polyethylene, and vinyl (**Fig. 2–28**). Powdered gloves rarely are used in blood collection because the glove powder can contaminate some tests and cause latex allergies as the latex particles are suspended in the air when gloves are removed. Allergy to latex is increasing among health-care workers. Persons developing symptoms of allergy to latex should avoid latex gloves and other latex products, such as tourniquets, at all times. Patients also may be allergic to latex. Be alert for signs stating this in the patients' rooms.

Antiseptics

The recommended antiseptic used for cleansing the skin in routine blood collection is 70 percent isopropyl alcohol. This is a bacteriostatic antiseptic used to prevent contamination by normal skin bacteria during the short period required to perform collection of the specimen. Individually wrapped prep pads are available for convenience.

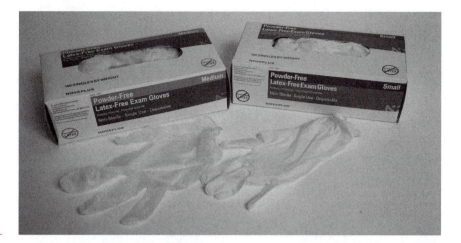

FIGURE 2–28. Gloves.

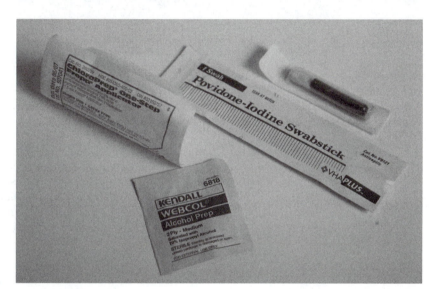

FIGURE 2–29. Antiseptics.

Iodine or chlorhexidine gluconate (for patients allergic to iodine) are used to cleanse the site for blood collections that require additional sterility, such as blood cultures and arterial punctures (**Fig. 2–29**). To prevent skin discomfort, iodine should always be removed from the patient's skin with alcohol after a collection procedure.

Gauze/Bandages

Clean 2 × 2–inch gauze pads are used for applying pressure to the puncture site immediately after the needle has been removed. Gauze pads also can provide additional pressure when folded in quarters and placed under a bandage. Cotton balls are not recommended because they stick to the site and disrupt the platelet plug when removed, which may reinitiate bleeding. Bandages or adhesive tape are placed over the puncture site when the bleeding has stopped. Self-adhesive gauze is preferred for patients who are allergic to adhesive bandages, the elderly with thin skin,

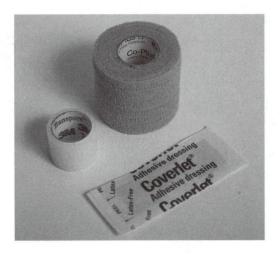

FIGURE 2–30. Bandages.

or when more pressure is required following arterial puncture or blood collection in patients with excessive bleeding. Latex-free bandages are available for patients with latex allergies. Patients should be instructed to remove the bandage within 1 hour (**Fig. 2–30**).

Additional Supplies

An essential piece of equipment is a pen for labeling tubes, initialing computer-generated labels, or noting unusual circumstances on the requisition form. Biohazard bags should be available for transport of specimens based on institutional protocol. Alcohol-based hand sanitizers are an acceptable substitute for hand washing when the hands are not visibly soiled. Wall-mounted hand sanitizers are available in all health-care settings in either gels or foams. Carrying personal bottles of hand sanitizers provides a convenient method of decontamination that is readily available (**Fig. 2–31**).

Quality Control

Ensuring the sterility of needles and puncture devices and the stability of evacuated tubes, anticoagulants, and additives is essential to patient safety and specimen quality. Disposable needles and puncture devices are individually packaged in tightly sealed sterile containers. Blood collectors should not use puncture equipment if the seal has been broken. Visual inspection for non-pointed or barbed needles may detect manufacturing defects.

Manufacturers of evacuated tubes must ensure that tubes, anticoagulants, and additives meet the standards established by the CLSI. Evacuated tubes produced at the same time are referred to as a lot and have a distinguishing lot number printed on the packages. There is also an expiration date printed on each package. The expiration date represents the last day the manufacturer guarantees the stability of the specified amount of vacuum in the tube and the reactivity of the anticoagulants and additives. The expiration date should be checked each time a new package of tubes is opened, and outdated tubes should not be used. Use of expired tubes may cause incompletely filled tubes (short draws), clotted anticoagulated specimens, improperly preserved specimens, and insecure gel barriers.

TECHNICAL TIP
Underfilled EDTA tubes cause red blood cell shrinkage, which will affect hematology tests.

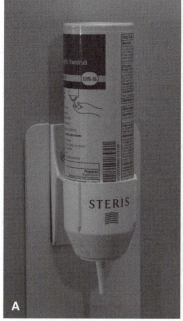 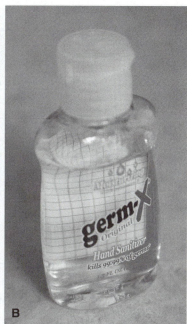

FIGURE 2–31. Hand sanitizers. *A,* Wall-mounted. *B,* Handheld.

TECHNICAL TIP

Avoid manual filling of additive tubes to maintain the correct blood to anti-coagulant ratio.

Failure to completely fill tubes (short draws) containing anticoagulants and additives affects specimen quality because the amount of anticoagulant or additive present in the tube is based on the assumption that the tube will be completely filled. Possible errors include excessive dilution of the specimen by liquid antico-agulants and distortion of cellular structures by increased chemical concentrations.

Venipuncture Equipment Selection Exercise

Instructions: State or assemble (if requested) the appropriate equipment for the following situations. Include the number and color of evacuated tubes; needle size, syringe size, or winged blood collection set, if appropri-ate. Instructors may specify the inclusion of supplies.

1. Collection of a CBC specimen from a 35-year-old woman.

_____

_____

_____

2. Collection of a CBC specimen from a 3-year-old boy.

_____

_____

_____

3. Collection of specimens for a CBC and electrolytes from a 40-year-old man.

_____
_____
_____

4. Collection of a cholesterol specimen from the hand of a patient.

_____
_____
_____

5. Collection of a specimen for a coagulation test from an elderly patient.

_____
_____
_____

6. Assemble the equipment to collect a specimen for a type and crossmatch on a 50-year-old man.

_____
_____
_____

7. Assemble the equipment to collect a specimen for a cardiac risk profile and a prothrombin time from a patient with fragile veins.

_____
_____
_____

REVIEW QUESTIONS

1. The possibility of hemolysis is increased with the use of a:
   a. 16-gauge needle
   b. 21-gauge needle
   c. 23-gauge needle
   d. 25-gauge needle

2. Pushing an evacuated tube through the stopper tube puncturing needle before entering the vein will result in:
   a. Collection of a hemolyzed specimen
   b. Quicker collection of the sample
   c. Inability to engage the safety device
   d. Failure to obtain the specimen

3. Upon completion of the blood collection, the holder is:
   a. Disinfected with hypochlorite
   b. Discarded in a different container than the needle
   c. Discarded with the needle attached
   d. Returned to the collection tray

4. Failure to gently and immediately mix an antico-agulated specimen will result in:
   a. Hemolysis
   b. Clot formation
   c. Loss of sterility
   d. Both a and b

5. Which of the following tubes will automatically be rejected by the laboratory if it is not completely filled?
   a. Light blue
   b. Gray
   c. Red/gray
   d. Light green

6. All of the following tubes contain separation gel EXCEPT:
   a. Gold Hemogard closure tubes
   b. Light green Hemogard closure tubes
   c. Red stopper tubes
   d. Red/gray rubber stopper tubes

7. You receive a requisition for the following tubes, light blue, lavender, yellow, and red. In what order should the tubes be drawn?
   a. Yellow, light blue, red, lavender
   b. Light blue, lavender, yellow, red
   c. Red, yellow, light blue, lavender
   d. Lavender, red, yellow, light blue

8. When transferring blood from a syringe to an evacuated tube, the recommended method is:
   a. Using a blood transfer device
   b. Puncturing the tube stopper
   c. Changing needles and puncturing the stopper
   d. Removing the tube stopper and the needle

9. The recommended antiseptic for routine venipuncture is:
   a. Chlorhexidine gluconate
   b. Isopropyl alcohol
   c. Antimicrobial soap
   d. Iodine

10. Using evacuated tubes past their expiration date may result in:
    a. Hemolyzed specimens
    b. Incompletely filled tubes
    c. Clotted anticoagulated tubes
    d. Both b and c

Internet Help

www.bd.com
www.gavenmedical.com
www.gbo.com
www.kendallhq.com
www.sarstedt.com
www.smiths-medical.com/
    brands/jelco

www.vacuette.com
www.vanishpoint.com
www.vascula.co.il
www.venoscope.com

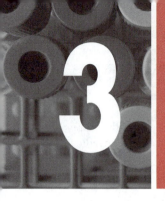

3

Routine Venipuncture

Introduction

The venipuncture technique consists of a series of steps that, when practiced consistently, provide quality specimens, and cause minimal patient discomfort. Administrative protocols vary among institutions, and, of course, every patient is different; however, many basic rules are the same in all situations. These basic rules must be followed to ensure the safety of the patient and the person performing the procedure and to produce specimens that are representative of the patient's condition.

This unit presents a detailed description of the recommended steps in the venipuncture procedure and possible complications that could occur at each step.

Blood Collection Procedure

Examine the Requisition Form

All blood collection procedures begin with the receipt of a test requisition form generated by or at the request of a health-care provider. The requisition is essential to provide the blood collector with the information needed to correctly identify the patient, organize the necessary equipment, collect the appropriate specimens, and provide legal protection. Blood specimens should not be collected without a requisition form, and this form must accompany the specimens sent to the laboratory.

The actual format of a requisition form may vary. Patient information may be handwritten or imprinted on color-coded forms with test check-off lists for different departments (**Fig. 3–1**). There may be multiple copies for purposes of record-keeping and billing. Computer-generated forms may include not only the patient information and tests requested but also the tube labels and bar codes for specimen processing, the number and type of collection tubes needed, and special collection instructions (**Fig. 3–2**). **Figure 3–3** shows an example of computer-generated labels.

When working in emergency care, a preprinted requisition form may not be available, making it necessary for the information to be written on a blank form. Be sure to transfer the identification number from the patient's wristband when a temporary identification system has been used. When verbal orders are given, the name of the person giving the order should be documented.

Requisitions must contain certain basic information to ensure that the specimen drawn and the test results are correlated to the appropriate patient and the results can be correctly interpreted

FIGURE 3–1. Manual requisition.

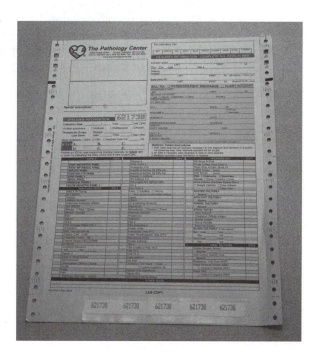

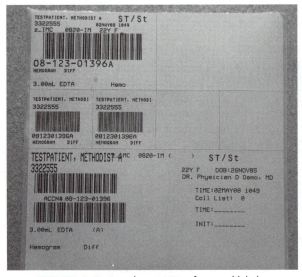

FIGURE 3-2. Sample requisition form and labels.

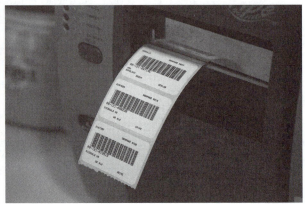

FIGURE 3-3. Computer labels printing in the laboratory.

with regard to any special conditions, such as the time of collection. The information includes the following:

1. Patient's name and identification number
2. Accession number
3. Patient's location
4. Health-care provider's name
5. Tests requested
6. Date and time of specimen collection

Other information that may be present includes:

- Patient's date of birth
- Special collection information (such as fasting specimen)
- Special patient information (such as areas that should not be used for venipuncture)
- Number and type of collection tubes
- Status of specimen (such as stat or timed)

TECHNICAL TIP

Personnel should never collect samples before the generation of a requisition form.

Greet the Patient

The blood collector should introduce himself or herself and ask permission to collect a blood specimen. This interaction begins the communication process and develops trust with the patient. The procedure must be explained in nontechnical terms and understood by the patient. The patient expects that the blood collector is competent in blood collection procedures. The patient is then able to give informed consent to the procedure. Consent may be verbal or non-verbal indicated by extending the arm or rolling up the sleeve. According to the Patient Bill of Rights, the patient has the right to refuse. The blood collector may be guilty of assault if the patient perceives that the blood collector is ignoring the refusal. Whenever possible, patients who are sleeping should be awakened and allowed to orient themselves prior to the procedure. The patient must be awake for accurate identification and to give informed consent for the procedure.

Unconscious patients should be greeted in the same manner as conscious patients, because they may be capable of hearing and understanding even though they cannot respond. In this circumstance, it may be necessary to request assistance from other members of the unit staff, because the patient may move when the needle is inserted.

Identify the Patient

The most important step in the venipuncture procedure is the correct identification of the patient. Serious diagnostic or treatment errors and even death can occur when blood is drawn from the wrong patient.

The Clinical and Laboratory Standards Institute (CLSI) recommends two identifiers for patient identification. The College of American Pathologists (CAP) and the Joint Commission (JC) patient safety goals require a minimum of two identifiers. To ensure that blood is drawn from the right patient, compare the information obtained verbally and from the patient's wrist identification (ID) band with the information on the requisition (**Fig. 3–4**). A wristband lying on the bedside table cannot be used for identification because it could belong to anyone. Likewise, a sign over the patient's bed or on the door cannot be relied on for identification because the patient could be in the wrong bed or room.

Verbal identification is made after the patient greeting by asking the patient to state his or her full name. In an outpatient setting, comparison of verbal information with the requisition form may be the only means of verifying identification. Asking a patient for his or her date of birth, address, or asking to spell his or her last name may be helpful in this situation. Do not ask, "Are you Mr. Jones?" because many patients will say "yes" to any questions asked. Verify that the computer-generated sample labels match the requisition and patient identification. The CLSI standard H3-A6 includes the requirement to compare the labeled specimen with the patient's identification bracelet or request the patient confirm the tube is properly labeled. This ensures that specimens are correctly labeled at the patient's bedside.

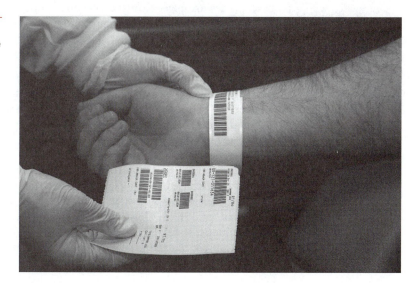

FIGURE 3–4. Identifying the patient by comparing the wrist ID band with the requisition.

For inpatients, examining the information on the patient's wristband, which should be present on all hospitalized patients, follows verbal identification. All information on the wrist ID band must match the information on the requisition form. The information should be identical, and any discrepancies investigated prior to obtaining the specimen. Positive patient identification can be made using bar-code technology. Using a wireless handheld computer, the blood collector positively identifies the patient by scanning the bar code on the patient's hospital ID band and the requisition form. After the patient has been properly identified, the specimen label is printed at the bedside by using a small portable wireless printer. The newest form of specimen identification is radio frequency identification (RFID). RFID tags are small silicon chips that transmit unique patient identification and specimen collection information obtained from the laboratory information system (LIS) to a wireless receiver. RFID tags are attached to the laboratory specimens and can be detected at various distances. The system tracks specimens as they are being transported to the laboratory.

Patients without ID bands attached to their bodies must have the band reapplied prior to specimen collection according to the institution's protocol. The name of the person identifying the patient should be documented. In the rare case that a patient cannot wear an ID band or there is not time to place the ID band, the nurse or caregiver must identify the patient and sign the requisition. If a patient is unable to properly identify himself or herself, the CLSI requires a caregiver or family member to provide identification information on the patient's behalf before blood collection. The name of the verifier must be documented. In the cases of drug testing, a photo ID might be required.

Unidentified patients are sometimes brought into the emergency room, and a system must be in place to ensure they are correctly matched with their laboratory work. The American Association of Blood Banks (AABB) requires that the patient is positively identified with a temporary but clear designation attached to the body. Some hospitals generate ID bands with an ID number and a tentative name, such as John Doe, or Patient X. The temporary ID must be placed on all requisitions and specimens and must be cross-referenced with the permanent identification name and number when it becomes available. Commercial identification systems are particularly useful when blood transfusions are required. In these systems, the ID band that is attached to the patient comes with matching identification stickers. The stickers are placed on the specimen tubes, the requisition form, and any units of blood designated for the patient. Blood bank identification systems are used in addition to routine ID bands, not instead of them.

SAFETY TIP

Personnel already familiar with a patient must never become lax with regard to patient identification.

Prepare and Position the Patient

The patient must be positioned conveniently and safely for the procedure. Provide a brief explanation of the procedure, but do not discuss the actual tests that are to be performed. Patients should not be told that the procedure will be painless. While talking with the patient, verify that any pretest preparation, such as fasting or abstaining from medications, has occurred. When these procedures have not been followed and the specimen is still required, the irregular condition, such as nonfasting, should be noted on the requisition form and on the specimen. Numerous variables associated with a patient's activities prior to specimen collection can affect the quality of the specimen. The ideal time to collect blood from a patient is when the patient is in a basal state. This is when the patient has refrained from strenuous exercise and has not ingested food or beverages except water for 12 hours. Normal values (reference values) for laboratory tests are determined from patients in a basal state to minimize the effects of preanalytical variables. These preanalytical variables can include diet, posture, exercise, stress,

TECHNICAL TIP

The College of American Pathologists recommends that drugs known to interfere with blood tests should be discontinued 4 to 24 hours before blood tests, and 48 to 72 hours before urine tests.

alcohol, smoking, time of day, and medications. Major tests affected by these variables are listed in **Table 3–1.** A variety of medications, both prescription and over-the-counter, can influence laboratory test results. Aspirin, medications that contain salicylate, and the use of certain herbs can interfere with platelet function or Coumadin anticoagulant therapy and may cause increased risk of bleeding. Common medications affecting laboratory tests are listed in **Table 3–2.** Physiologic variables, such as age, altitude, and gender affect normal values for test results. Other patient conditions that will influence laboratory test results are dehydration, fever, and pregnancy.

To guard against a possible episode of syncope, patients should always be sitting or lying down when phlebotomy is performed. Never draw blood from a patient who is standing. Outpatients are seated or reclined in a drawing chair, preferably one with a movable arm that serves the dual purpose of providing a solid surface for the patient's arm and preventing a patient who faints from falling out of the chair. Patients who have had previous difficulties during venipuncture should lie down for the procedure. When collecting a blood specimen from a patient in a home setting, the patient must be seated in a chair with armrests and the patient's arm placed on a hard surface. A sofa or bed may be used if the patient is anxious or has had previous difficulties during venipuncture. Placing a pillow or towel under the patient's arm can provide comfortable support. Asking the patient to make a fist with the opposite hand and placing it behind the elbow will provide support. The arm should be firmly supported and extended downward in a straight line, allowing the tube to fill from the bottom up to prevent reflux and anticoagulant carryover between sample tubes (**Fig. 3–5**).

TABLE 3–1. Major Tests Affected by Patient Variables

VARIABLE	INCREASED RESULTS	DECREASED RESULTS
Nonfasting	Glucose and triglycerides	
Prolonged fasting	Bilirubin, fatty acids, and triglycerides	Glucose
Posture	Albumin, aldosterone, bilirubin, calcium, cholesterol, enzymes, iron, total protein, triglycerides, renin, RBCs, and WBCs	
Short-term exercise	Creatinine, fatty acids, glucose, insulin, lactate, protein AST, CK, LD, and WBCs	Arterial pH, PCO_2
Long-term exercise	Aldolase, creatinine, sex hormones, AST, CK, and LD	
Stress	Adrenal hormones, fatty acids, lactate, and WBCs	Serum iron
Alcohol	Lactate, triglycerides, uric acid, GGT, HDL, and MCV	
Tobacco	Catecholamines, cholesterol, cortisol, glucose, hemoglobin, IgE, MCV, triglyceride, and WBCs	Immunoglobulins IgA, IgG, and IgM
Diurnal variation (AM)	Bilirubin, cortisol, hemoglobin, insulin, potassium, renin, serum iron, testosterone, RBCs, TSH	Creatinine, eosinophils, glucose, phosphate, triglyceride
Dehydration	Calcium, coagulation factors, enzymes, iron, RBCs, sodium	
Fever	Cortisol, glucagons, insulin	
Pregnancy		RBCs

AST, aspartate aminotransferase; CK, creatine kinase; GGT, gamma-glutamyl transpeptidase; HDL, high-density lipoprotein; LD, lactate dehydrogenase; IgE, immunoglobulin E; MCV, mean corpuscular volume; RBCs, red blood cells; WBCs, white blood cells; TSH, thyroid stimulating hormone

TABLE 3–2. Common Medications Affecting Laboratory Tests

MEDICATION	AFFECTED TESTS/SYSTEMS
Acetaminophen and certain antibiotics	Elevated liver enzymes and bilirubin
Cholesterol-lowering drugs	Prolonged PT and APTT
Certain antibiotics	Elevated BUN, creatinine, and electrolyte imbalance
Corticosteroids and estrogen	Elevated amylase and lipase
Diuretics	Increased calcium, glucose, and uric acid
Chemotherapy	Decreased RBCs, WBCs, and platelets
Aspirin, salicylates, and herbal supplements	Prolonged PT and bleeding time
Radiographic contrast media	Routine urinalysis
Fluorescein dye	Increased creatinine, cortisol, and digoxin

BUN, blood urea nitrogen.

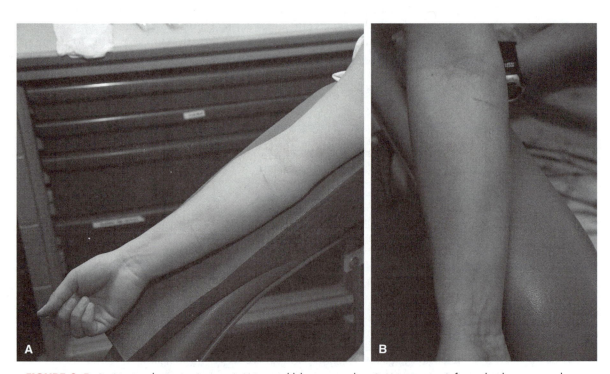

FIGURE 3–5. Positioning the patient's arm. *A,* Using a phlebotomy wedge. *B,* Using patient's fist under the arm as a brace.

A patient should remove any foreign object, such as food, drink, gum, or a thermometer, from his or her mouth before performance of the venipuncture. Always ask the patient if he or she is allergic to latex.

Some patients may refuse to have their blood drawn, and they have the right to do this. If the patient refuses, this decision should be documented according to the institution policy.

Select Equipment

Before approaching the patient for the actual venipuncture, the blood collector should collect all necessary supplies (including collection equipment, antiseptic pads, gauze pads, bandages, and needle disposal system) and place them close to the patient. The blood collection tray should not be placed on the bed or on the patient's eating table. Place supplies on the same side as your free hand during blood collection to avoid reaching across the patient and causing unnecessary movement of the needle in the patient's vein. Reexamine the requisition form, and select the appropriate number and type of collection tubes. Check the expiration date on each tube and discard any tube that is beyond its expiration date. Place the tubes in the correct order for specimen collection, and have additional tubes readily available for possible use during the procedure (**Fig. 3–6**). It is not uncommon to find an evacuated tube that does not contain the necessary amount of vacuum to collect a full tube of blood. Accidentally pushing a tube past the indicator mark on the holder before the vein is entered also results in loss of vacuum.

Wash Hands and Apply Gloves

Always apply clean gloves between each patient, and wash hands before and after the procedure. Pull gloves over the cuffs of protective clothing.

Apply the Tourniquet

The tourniquet serves two functions in the venipuncture procedure. By causing blood to accumulate in the veins, the tourniquet causes the veins to be more easily located and also provides a larger amount of blood for collection. Use of a tourniquet can alter some test results by increasing the ratio of cellular elements to plasma (hemoconcentration) and by causing hemolysis. Therefore, the maximum time a tourniquet should remain in place is 1 minute.

FIGURE 3–6. Venipuncture collection equipment.

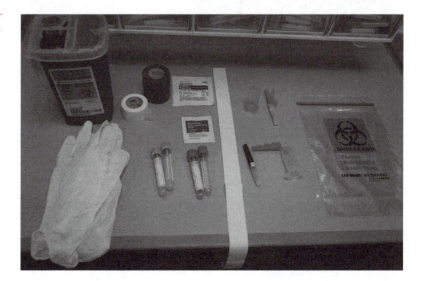

This may require that the tourniquet be applied twice during the venipuncture procedure; first when vein selection is being made and then immediately before the puncture is performed. When the tourniquet is used during vein selection, it should be released for 2 minutes before being reapplied.

Tests most likely to be affected by prolonged tourniquet application are those measuring large molecules, such as plasma proteins and lipids, or analytes affected by hemolysis, including potassium, lactic acid, and enzymes. During multiple tube collections, the tourniquet must be removed when the timing exceeds 1 minute. Tourniquet application and fist clenching are not recommended when drawing specimens for lactic acid determinations.

Other causes of hemoconcentration are excessive squeezing or probing a site, long-term IV therapy, sclerosed or occluded veins, and vigorous fist clenching. **Box 3–1** lists the major tests affected by hemoconcentration.

Ideally, the tourniquet should be released as soon as blood begins to flow into the first tube to prevent hemoconcentration and hemolysis. Difficulty filling additional tubes may be encountered, however; the tourniquet may have to be retightened or pressure applied to the area with the free hand to increase the amount of blood present in the vein.

The tourniquet should be placed on the arm 3 to 4 inches above the venipuncture site. Application of the tourniquet (preferably single-use, latex-free) requires practice to develop a smooth technique and can be difficult if properly fitting gloves are not worn. **Figure 3–7** shows the technique used for tourniquet application. To achieve adequate pressure, both sides of the tourniquet must be grasped near the patient's arm, and while maintaining tension, the left side is tucked under the right side. The loop formed should face downward. The free ends of the tourniquet must be pointing away from the venipuncture site to avoid contaminating the site and must be able to be easily released with one hand. Left-handed persons would reverse this procedure.

Tourniquets that are folded or applied too tightly are uncomfortable for the patient and may obstruct blood flow to the area. The appearance of small, reddish discolorations (petechiae) on the patient's arm, blanching of the skin around the tourniquet, and the blood collector's inability to feel a radial pulse are indications of a tourniquet tied too tightly.

When dealing with patients with skin conditions or open sores, it may be necessary to place the tourniquet over the patient's gown or to cover the area with gauze prior to application. If possible, another area should be selected for the venipuncture. Do not apply a tourniquet to an arm on the same side as a mastectomy.

Select the Venipuncture Site

The preferred site for venipuncture is the antecubital fossa located anterior to the elbow. As shown in **Figure 3–8**, the median cubital, cephalic, and basilic veins are located in this area, and in most patients at least one of these veins can

TECHNICAL TIP

When supporting the patient's arm, do not hyperextend the elbow. This may make vein palpation difficult. Sometimes bending the elbow very slightly may aid in vein palpation.

BOX 3–1. Tests Affected by Hemoconcentration

Albumin	Lactic acid
Ammonia	Lipids
Bilirubin	Potassium
Calcium	Proteins
Enzymes	Red blood cells
Iron	

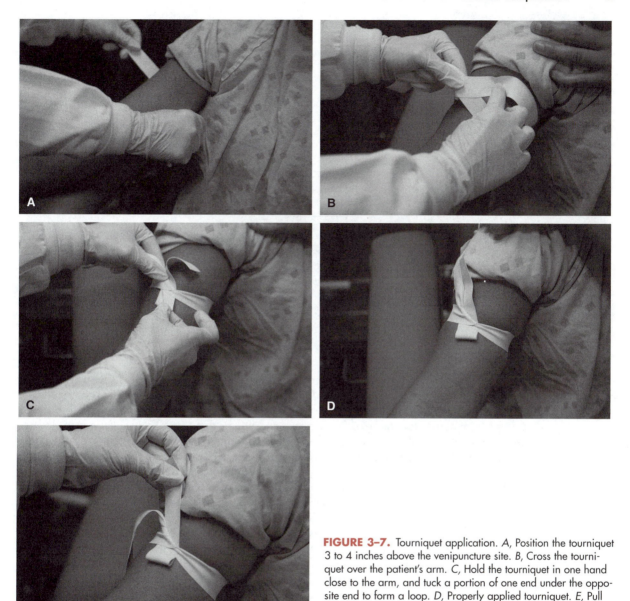

FIGURE 3–7. Tourniquet application. *A,* Position the tourniquet 3 to 4 inches above the venipuncture site. *B,* Cross the tourniquet over the patient's arm. *C,* Hold the tourniquet in one hand close to the arm, and tuck a portion of one end under the opposite end to form a loop. *D,* Properly applied tourniquet. *E,* Pull end of loop to release tourniquet.

be easily located. Notice that the veins continue down the forearm to the wrist area; however, in these areas the veins become smaller and less well anchored, and punctures are more painful to the patient. Small, prominent veins are also located in the back of the hand. When necessary, these veins can be used for venipuncture but may require a smaller needle or winged blood collection set. The veins of the lower arm and hand are also the preferred sites for administering IV fluids because they allow the patient more arm flexibility. Frequent venipuncture in these veins could make them unsuitable for IV use. Some institutions have special ID bands that indicate the restricted use of veins being used for other procedures.

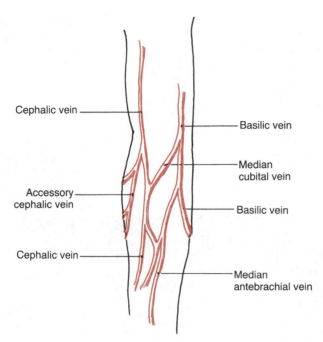

Cephalic vein

Basilic vein

Median
cubital vein

Accessory
cephalic vein

Basilic vein

Cephalic vein

Median
antebrachial vein

FIGURE 3–8. The veins in the arm most often chosen for venipuncture *(From Strasinger, SK, and Di Lorenzo, MS: The Phlebotomy Workbook. FA Davis, Philadelphia, 2003, Figure 6–8, p. 119, with permission.*

Of the three veins located in the antecubital area, the median cubital is the vein of choice because it is large, well anchored, and does not tend to move when the needle is inserted. It is often closer to the surface of the skin, more isolated from underlying structures, and the least painful to puncture as there are fewer nerve endings in this area. The cephalic vein, located on the thumb side of the arm, is usually more difficult to locate, except possibly in larger patients, and has more tendency to move. Because this vein is closer to the surface, there is the possibility of a blood spurt when the needle is inserted into the vein. This often is controlled by decreasing the angle of needle insertion to 15 degrees. The cephalic vein should be the second choice if the median cubital is inaccessible in both arms. The basilic vein should be used as the last choice because the median nerve and brachial artery are in close proximity to it, increasing the risk of injury. The basilic vein is the least firmly anchored; therefore, it has a tendency to roll and hematoma formation is more likely. Using a syringe method for blood collection from the basilic vein offers more control over a rolling vein. The basilic vein is located near the brachial artery and extreme care must be taken not to accidentally puncture the artery. The CLSI standard H3-A6 recommends locating the brachial pulse before accessing the basilic vein. Only superficial veins should be used in children.

Two routine steps in the venipuncture procedure aid in locating a suitable vein: applying a tourniquet and asking the patient to clench his or her fist. Continuous clenching or pumping of the fist is not recommended because it will result in hemoconcentration, altering some test results, such as potassium and ionized calcium. The tourniquet can be applied for only 1 minute; therefore, after the vein is located, the tourniquet should be removed while the site is being cleansed, and then reapplied immediately before the venipuncture.

Veins are located by sight and touch, referred to as palpation. The ability to feel a vein is much more important than the ability to see a vein. Palpation

TECHNICAL TIP

Patients often think they are helping by pumping their fists, because this is an acceptable practice when donating blood. In contrast to laboratory specimens, a donated unit of blood is even better when it is hemoconcentrated.

is performed by using the tip of the index finger to probe the antecubital area with a pushing rather than a stroking motion. Feel for the vein in both a vertical and horizontal direction. Gloves should be worn when palpating veins to prevent contact with microorganisms, such as methicillin-resistant *Staphylococcus aureus* (MRSA) and vancomycin-resistant enterococci (VRE); however, the CLSI standard H3-A6 does permit gloves to be applied just prior to site preparation instead of prior to locating the vein.

TECHNICAL TIP

Using the nondominant hand for palpation may be helpful when additional palpation is to be done immediately before performing the puncture.

Palpation is used to determine the size, depth, and direction of the vein to aid in directing the needle during insertion. The pressure applied by palpating locates deep veins and distinguishes veins, which feel like spongy cords, from rigid tendon cords. Veins must be differentiated from arteries, which produce a pulse; therefore, the thumb should not be used to palpate because it has a pulse beat. Select a vein that is easily palpated and large enough to support good blood flow (**Fig. 3–9**). It is often helpful to find a visual reference for the selected vein, such as a mole, freckle, or skin crease, to assist in relocating the vein after cleansing the site. Many patients have prominent veins in one arm and not in the other arm. Checking the patient's other arm should be the first thing done when a site is not easily located. Patients with veins that are difficult to locate often point out areas of previously successful venipunctures. Palpation of these areas may prove beneficial and is also good for patient relations.

Other techniques to enhance the prominence of veins include massaging the arm upward from the wrist to the elbow, briefly hanging the arm down, and applying heat to the site. A transilluminator device is helpful for locating veins, particularly in children. Remember that the tourniquet should not remain tied for more than 1 minute at a time when performing these techniques.

If no palpable veins are found in the antecubital area, the wrist and the back of the hand should be examined. The tourniquet should be retied on the forearm. Because the veins in these areas are smaller, it may be necessary to change equipment and use a smaller needle with a syringe, a winged blood collection set, or a smaller evacuated tube. CLSI standard H3-A6 cautions against selecting veins on the underside of the wrists to prevent nerve and tendon injuries.

Veins in the legs and feet are sometimes used as venipuncture sites. They should be used only with physician approval. Leg veins are more susceptible to infection and the formation

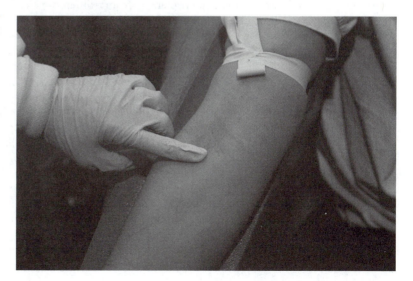

FIGURE 3–9. Palpating for a vein using the fingers, not the thumb.

of clots (thrombi), particularly in patients with diabetes, cardiac problems, and coagulation disorders.

Veins that contain thrombi or that have been subjected to numerous venipunctures often feel hard (sclerosed) and should be avoided because they may be blocked (occluded) and have impaired circulation. Areas that appear blue or are cold also may have impaired circulation.

The presence of a hematoma indicates that blood has accumulated in the tissue surrounding a vein. Puncturing into a hematoma not only is painful for the patient but also results in the collection of old, hemolyzed blood from the hematoma rather than from circulating venous blood that is representative of the patient's current condition. If a vein containing a hematoma must be used, blood should be collected below the hematoma to ensure sampling of free-flowing blood. Drawing from areas containing excess tissue fluid (edema) also is not recommended because the sample will be contaminated with tissue fluid.

Extensively burned and scarred areas, including areas with tattoos, are more susceptible to infection; they also have decreased circulation and veins that are difficult to palpate.

Applying a tourniquet or drawing blood from an arm located on the same side of the body as a mastectomy can be harmful to the patient and produce erroneous test results. Removal of lymph nodes as part of the mastectomy procedure interferes with the flow of lymph fluid (lymphostasis) and increases the blood level of lymphocytes and waste products normally contained in the lymph fluid. Patients are in danger of developing lymphedema in the affected area. The protective functions of the lymphatic system are also lost, so that the area becomes more prone to infection. For these reasons, blood should be drawn from the other arm or possibly from the hand. In the case of a double mastectomy, the physician should be consulted as to an appropriate site. It may be possible to perform the tests from a finger stick.

When a patient is receiving IV fluids, blood should be drawn from the other arm. Whenever possible, areas near the site of a previous IV should be avoided for 24 to 48 hours. When a patient has IVs in both arms, it is preferable to collect the specimen by dermal puncture if possible. If an arm containing an IV must be used for specimen collection, the site selected must be below the IV insertion point and preferably from a different vein. A nurse may choose to collect blood from an IV line that is inserted into the vein. The IV should be turned off for at least 2 minutes and the first 5 mL of blood drawn must be discarded because it may be contaminated with IV fluid.

When using a syringe, a new syringe must be used for the specimen collection. If a coagulation test is ordered, an additional 5 mL of blood (total of 10 mL) should be drawn before collecting the coagulation test specimen, because IV lines are frequently flushed with heparin. This additional blood can be used for other tests, if they have been ordered. When blood is collected from an arm containing an IV, the type of fluid and location must be noted on the requisition form. Avoid collecting blood too soon after dye for a radiological procedure has been injected or when a unit of blood is being infused.

Patients receiving renal dialysis have a permanent surgical fusion of an artery and a vein called a fistula in one arm, and this arm should be avoided for venipuncture because of the possibility of infection. The dialysis patient also may have a temporary external connection between the artery and a vein formed by a cannula that contains a special T-tube connector with a diaphragm for drawing blood. Only specifically trained personnel are authorized to draw blood from a cannula. Be sure to check for the presence of a fistula or cannula before applying

TECHNICAL TIP

Never be reluctant to check both arms and to listen to the patient's suggestions.

TECHNICAL TIP

According to the CLSI standard H3-A6, an attempt must have been made to locate the median cubital vein on both arms before considering other veins.

TECHNICAL TIP

Most mastectomy patients have been told never to have blood drawn from the affected side. Make sure they receive appropriate reassurance if an alternate site is not available and use of the affected side has been approved.

a tourniquet to the arm, because this can compromise the patient. Accidental puncture of the area around the fistula can cause prolonged bleeding.

Cleanse the Site

After the vein is located, release the tourniquet and cleanse the site using a 70-percent isopropyl alcohol prep pad. Use a circular motion starting at the inside of the venipuncture site and work outward in widening concentric circles (**Fig. 3–10**). Repeat this procedure for dirty skin. For maximum bacteriostatic action to occur, the alcohol should be allowed to dry for 30 to 60 seconds on the patient's arm rather than being wiped off with a gauze pad. Performing a venipuncture before the alcohol has dried causes a stinging sensation for the patient and may hemolyze the specimen. Do not reintroduce contaminants by blowing on the site, fanning the area, drying the site with unsterile gauze, or touching the site after cleansing it. If additional palpation of the vein is needed after the cleansing process, the phlebotomist should use alcohol to cleanse the gloved end of the finger to be used and touch only above or below the needle insertion point.

Blood cultures and arterial blood gases require that the site be cleansed with an antiseptic stronger than isopropyl alcohol. The most frequently used solutions are povidone-iodine, tincture of iodine, or chlorhexidine gluconate, which is used for persons allergic to iodine.

Alcohol should not be used to cleanse the site prior to drawing a blood alcohol level. Thoroughly cleansing the site with soap and water ensures the least amount of interference, and some institutions find iodine or benzalkonium chloride (Zephiran Chloride) to be acceptable.

Examine and Assemble Puncture Equipment

While the alcohol is drying, make a final survey of the supplies at hand to be sure everything required for the procedure is present, and assemble the equipment.

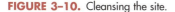

FIGURE 3–10. Cleansing the site.

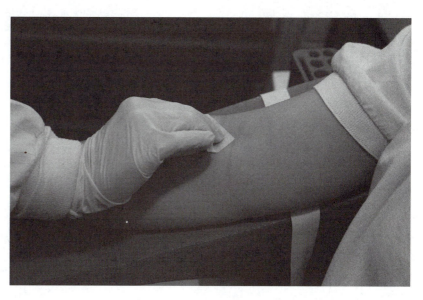

Screw the stopper-puncturing end of the double-ended evacuated tube needle into the needle holder. Do not remove the sterile cap from the other end of the needle. Insert the first tube to be collected into the needle holder up to the designated mark. After the tube is pushed up to the mark, it may retract slightly when pressure is released. This is acceptable.

Perform the Venipuncture

Reapply the tourniquet and confirm the puncture site. If necessary, cleanse the gloved palpating finger for additional vein palpation. Ask the patient to again make a fist.

The needle holder or syringe is held securely in the dominant hand with the thumb on top and the other fingers below. Before entering the vein, remove the needle's plastic cap and visually examine the point of the needle for any defects, such as a nonpointed or rough (barbed) end. Position the needle for entry into the vein with the bevel facing up.

Use the thumb of the nondominant hand to anchor the selected vein while inserting the needle (**Fig. 3–11A**). Place the thumb 1 or 2 inches below and slightly to the side of the insertion site, and the four fingers on the back of the arm and pull the skin taut. Anchoring the vein above and below the site using the thumb and index finger is not an acceptable technique, because sudden patient movement could cause the index finger to be punctured. A vein that moves to the side is said to have "rolled." Patients often state that they have "rolling veins"; however, all veins will roll if they are not properly anchored. These patients are really saying that they have had blood drawn by practitioners who were not anchoring the veins well enough. As mentioned previously, the median cubital vein is the easiest to anchor and the basilic vein is the most difficult. In general, the closer a vein is to the surface, the more likely it is to roll.

When the vein is securely anchored, align the needle with the vein and insert it, bevel up, at an angle of 15 to 30 degrees depending on the depth of the vein (**Fig. 3–11B**). It should be done in a smooth quick movement so the patient feels the stick only briefly. You will notice a feeling of lessening of resistance to the needle movement when the vein has been entered. After needle insertion is made, the fingers are braced against the patient's arm to provide stability while tubes are being changed in the holder, or the plunger of the syringe is being pulled back. **Figure 3–11** provides additional illustration of the venipuncture procedure.

Once the vein has been entered, the hand anchoring the vein can be moved and used to push the evacuated tube completely into the holder or to pull back on the syringe plunger (**Fig. 3–11C**). Use the thumb to push the tube onto the back of the evacuated tube needle, while the index and middle fingers grasp the flared ends of the holder. Blood should begin to flow into the tube and the tourniquet can be released (**Fig. 3–11D**), although if the procedure does not last more than 1 minute, the tourniquet can be left on until the last tube is filled. Ask the patient to relax his or her fist. Some practitioners prefer to change hands at this point so that the dominant hand is free for performing the remaining tasks. Changing hands is usually better suited for use by experienced persons, because holding the needle steady in the patient's vein is often difficult for beginners.

The hand used to hold the needle assembly should remain braced on the patient's arm. This is of particular importance when evacuated tubes are being inserted or removed from the holder, because a certain amount of resistance is encountered and can cause the needle to be pushed through or pulled out of the vein. Tubes should be gently twisted on and off the puncturing needle using the flared ends of the holder as an additional brace (**Fig. 3–11E**).

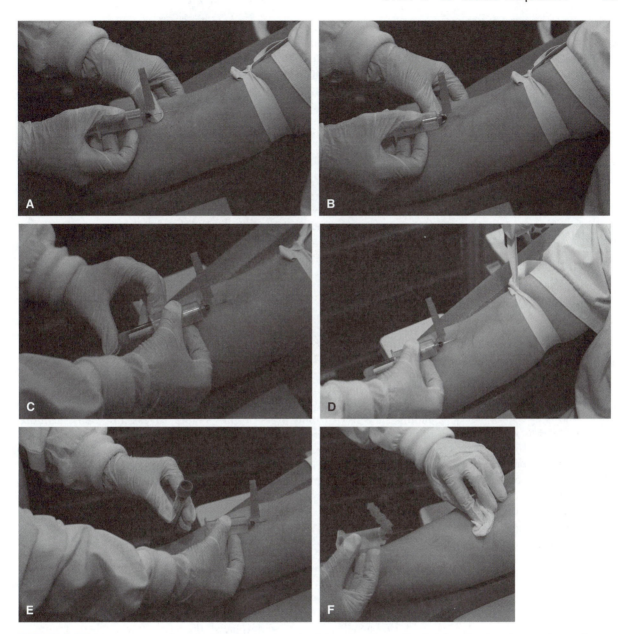

FIGURE 3–11. Venipuncture technique. *A*, Anchoring the vein. *B*, Inserting the needle. *C*, Advancing the tube onto the needle. *D*, Removing the tourniquet. *E*, Removing the last tube and preparing to mix the tube. *F*, Appling pressure.

To prevent any chance of blood refluxing back into the needle, tubes should be held at a downward angle while they are being filled and have slight pressure applied to them. Be sure to follow the prescribed order of draw when multiple tubes are being collected, and allow the tubes to fill completely before removing them. Mixing of evacuated tubes by gentle inversion 3 to 8 times depending on the anticoagulant or additive should be done as soon as the tube is removed and before another tube is placed in the assembly. The few seconds required does not cause additional discomfort to the patient and ensures that the specimen will be acceptable. Delay in mixing the specimen may cause clots to form and necessitate recollecting the specimen.

When the last tube has been filled, it is removed from the assembly and mixed prior to completing the procedure. Failure to remove the evacuated tube before removing the needle causes blood to drip from the end of the needle, resulting in unnecessary contamination and possible damage to the patient's clothes.

Remove the Needle

Before removing the needle, remove the tourniquet by pulling on the free end. Failure to remove the tourniquet before removing the needle may produce a hematoma.

Fold the gauze into fourths and place over the venipuncture site, smoothly withdraw the needle, and apply pressure to the site as soon as the needle is withdrawn (**Fig. 3–11F**). Do not apply pressure while the needle is still in the vein. To prevent blood from leaking into the surrounding tissue and producing a hematoma, pressure must be applied until the bleeding has stopped. The arm should be held in a raised, outstretched position. Bending the elbow to apply pressure allows blood to leak into the tissue more easily, causing a hematoma. A capable patient can be asked to apply the pressure, thereby freeing the blood collector to dispose of the used needle and label the specimen tubes. If this is not possible, the blood collector must apply the pressure and perform the other tasks after the bleeding has stopped.

Dispose of the Contaminated Needle

On completion of the venipuncture, the contaminated needle with safety device activated must be disposed of immediately in an approved sharps container conveniently located near the patient (**Figs. 3–12A and B**). As discussed in Unit 2, the method by which this is done depends on the type of disposal equipment selected by the institution. Under no circumstance should the needle be bent, cut, placed on a counter or bed, manually recapped, or removed from the tube holder after use.

Label the Tubes

Tubes must be labeled at the time of specimen collection, before leaving the patient's room or dismissing an outpatient. Tubes are labeled by writing with an indelible pen on the attached label or by applying a computer-generated label (**Figs. 3–13A and B**). Tubes should not be labeled before the specimen is collected, because this can result in confusion of specimens when more than

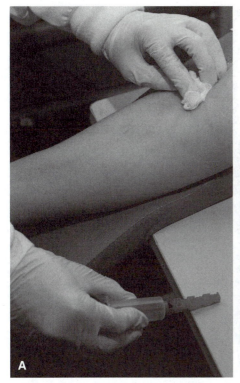

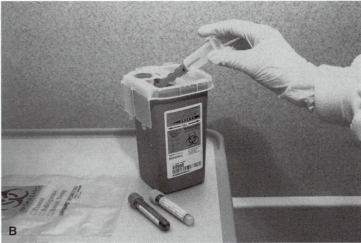

FIGURE 3–12. Needle disposal. *A,* Activating safety shield. *B,* Safety shield activated and disposal of safety needle and holder.

one patient is having blood drawn or when a specimen cannot be collected. Preprinted labels should be verified before being attached to the specimen. Compare the labeled specimen to the patient's ID band or request the patient confirm that the tube is correctly labeled (**Fig. 3–13***C*). Mislabeled specimens, just like misidentified patients, can result in serious patient harm.

Information on the specimen label should include:

- Patient's name and ID number
- Date and time of collection
- Collector's initials

Additional information may be present on computer-generated labels. The laboratory will reject incompletely and unlabeled tubes. Specimens for blood bank may require an additional label obtained from the patient's blood bank ID band.

Specimens requiring special handling, such as cooling or warming, are placed in the appropriate container when labeling is complete.

Bandage the Patient's Arm

Bleeding at the venipuncture site should stop within 5 minutes. Before applying the bandage, the blood collector should examine the patient's arm to be sure the bleeding has stopped. For additional pressure, an adhesive bandage or paper tape is applied over a folded-gauze square

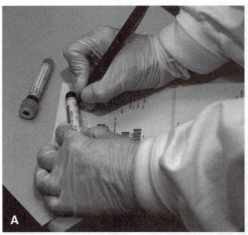
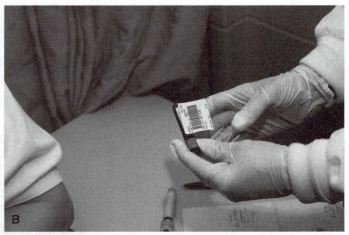
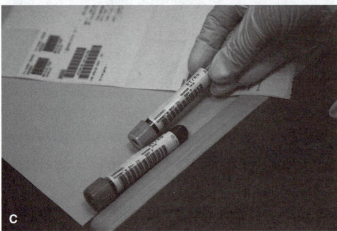

FIGURE 3–13. Labeling the tube. *A,* Handwriting a label. *B,* Applying computer label to a tube. *C,* Verifying preprinted labels.

(**Fig. 3–14***A*). The patient should be instructed to remove the bandage within 1 hour to avoid irritation and to avoid using the arm to carry heavy objects during that period.

Patients receiving anticoagulant medications or large amounts of aspirin or herbs or patients with coagulation disorders may continue to bleed after pressure has been applied for 5 minutes. **Box 3–2** lists the herbs affecting coagulation testing. Continue to apply pressure until the bleeding has stopped. A self-adhering gauze-like material, such as a CoBan dressing, can be used (**Fig. 3–14***B*).

In the case of an accidental arterial puncture, which usually can be detected by the appearance of unusually red blood that spurts into the tube, the blood collector, not the patient, should apply pressure to the site for 10 minutes. The fact that the specimen is arterial blood should be recorded on the requisition form.

Some patients are allergic to adhesive bandages, and it may be necessary to wrap gauze around the arm prior to applying the adhesive tape. Bandages are not recommended for children younger than 2 years old, because children may put bandages in their mouth.

SAFETY TIP

The practice of quickly applying tape over the gauze without checking the puncture site frequently produces hematomas.

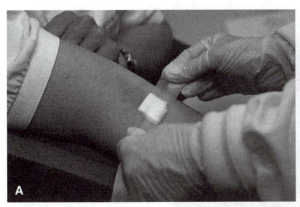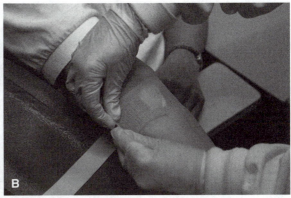

FIGURE 3–14. Patient's arm with bandage. *A*, Using an adhesive bandage. *B*, Using self-adhering material (Co-Ban).

BOX 3–2. Herbs Having Effects on Coagulation	
Chamomile	Ginseng
Clove	Goldenseal
Echinacea	Horse Chestnut
Evening primrose oil	Kava Kava
Feverfew	Licorice
Garlic	Meadowsweet
Ginger	Poplar
Ginkgo biloba	White willow

Dispose of Used Supplies

Before leaving the patient's room, dispose of all contaminated supplies, such as alcohol, pads, and gauze in a biohazard container; remove gloves and dispose of them in the biohazard container; and wash your hands.

Thank the Patient

Patients should be thanked for their cooperation in both inpatient and outpatient settings. Leave the patient's room in the condition in which you found it (bed and bedrails in the same position).

Deliver Specimens to the Laboratory

Use designated biohazard containers for transport, and securely attach the requisitions with the specimen (**Fig. 3–15**). Specimens must be delivered to the laboratory as soon as possible. Gently transport specimens in a vertical position to facilitate clotting and prevent hemolysis.

Specimen Processing

The stability of analytes varies greatly, as do the accepted methods of preservation. This is why rapid delivery to the laboratory or following laboratory prescribed specimen handling protocols is essential. Common protocols include separation of the plasma or serum from the cells (either

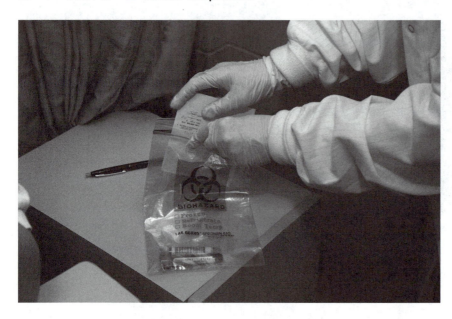

FIGURE 3–15. Placing specimen and requisition in a biohazard bag for transporting.

manually or by gel), storage temperature, and protecting the specimen from exposure to light. Gel separation tubes must always be stored in an upright position.

The CLSI recommends centrifugation of tubes and the separation of plasma or serum from the cells within 2 hours. Ideally, the specimen should reach the laboratory within 45 minutes and be centrifuged on arrival. Tests most frequently affected by improper processing include glucose, potassium, and coagulation tests. Glycolysis caused by the use of glucose in cellular metabolism causes falsely lower glucose values. Hemolysis and leakage of intracellular potassium into the serum or plasma falsely elevates potassium results. Coagulation factors are very labile, therefore, for optimal results, specimens for coagulation testing should be delivered to the laboratory for testing within ½ hour of collection. Logistically this is not always possible. According to the CLSI guidelines, coagulation specimens for activated partial thromboplastin times (APTTs) are stable at room temperature for 4 hours unless the patient is on heparin, in which case, the plasma must be removed from the cells within 1 hour after collection and tested within 4 hours. Specimens for pro-thrombin time (PT) testing are stable for 24 hours at room temperature. All other coagulation tests must be performed with 4 hours of collection. When samples cannot be assayed within the required time frame, the plasma must be separated from the red cells and frozen within 1 hour of collection. Lavender stopper tubes should be refrigerated if testing is not performed within 4 hours. Appendix C summarizes the requirements of some routinely encountered analytes.

The venipuncture procedure is complete when the specimen is delivered to the laboratory in satisfactory condition and all appropriate paperwork has been completed. These procedures vary, depending on institutional protocol and the types of specimens collected.

TECHNICAL TIP

Verification of the specimen collection either into the computer or recorded in a logbook completes the collection process.

Summary of Venipuncture Technique Using an Evacuated Tube System

1. Obtain and examine the requisition form.
2. Greet the patient.
3. Identify the patient.
4. Reassure the patient and explain the procedure.
5. Prepare the patient.
6. Select supplies and puncturing equipment.
7. Wash hands and apply gloves.
8. Apply the tourniquet.
9. Select the venipuncture site.
10. Release the tourniquet.
11. Cleanse the site.
12. Assemble equipment.
13. Reapply the tourniquet.
14. Confirm the venipuncture site.
15. Examine the needle.
16. Anchor the vein.
17. Insert the needle.
18. Push evacuated tube completely into holder.
19. Gently invert the specimens, as they are collected.
20. Remove last tube from the holder.
21. Release the tourniquet.
22. Place gauze over the needle.
23. Remove the needle, and apply pressure.
24. Activate needle safety device.
25. Dispose of the needle with the safety device activated and attached to the holder.
26. Label the tubes and confirm with the patient or ID band.
27. Perform appropriate specimen handling.
28. Examine the patient's arm.
29. Bandage the patient's arm.
30. Dispose of used supplies.
31. Remove and dispose of gloves.
32. Wash hands.
33. Thank the patient.
34. Complete any required paperwork.
35. Deliver specimens to appropriate locations.

Venipuncture Situation Exercises

1. Determine if the following are acceptable or not acceptable when performing a venipuncture, and explain your reason in one sentence.

   a. An outpatient with a sore back wishes to stand during the procedure.

   _____

   b. Assembling equipment before applying the tourniquet.

   _____

   c. Requesting the patient to pump his or her fist during sample collection.

   _____

   d. Cleansing the site in a circular motion from inside to outside.

   _____

   e. Bending the patient's elbow while applying pressure to the puncture site.

   _____

2. State an error in routine venipuncture technique that may cause:

   a. A hematoma

   _____

   b. Petechiae

   _____

   c. A patient to choke

   _____

   d. Blood to stop flowing when a tube is changed

   _____

   e. Blood drops on a patient's slacks when the needle is removed

   _____

Evaluation of Venipuncture Technique Using an Evacuated Tube System

Rating System   **2 = Satisfactory**   **1 = Needs Improvement**   **0 = Incorrect/Did Not Perform**

_____ 1. Examines requisition form.
_____ 2. Greets patient and states procedure to be done.
_____ 3. Identifies the patient verbally.
_____ 4. Examines patient's ID band.
_____ 5. Compares requisition information with ID band.

_____ 6. Selects correct tubes and equipment for procedure.
_____ 7. Washes hands and puts on gloves.
_____ 8. Positions patient's arm.
_____ 9. Applies tourniquet.
_____ 10. Identifies vein by palpation.
_____ 11. Releases tourniquet.

_____ 12. Cleanses site and allows it to air dry.
_____ 13. Assembles equipment.
_____ 14. Reapplies tourniquet.
_____ 15. Does not touch puncture site with unclean finger.
_____ 16. Examines needle.
_____ 17. Anchors vein below puncture site.
_____ 18. Smoothly enters vein at appropriate angle with bevel up.
_____ 19. Does not move needle when changing tubes.
_____ 20. Collects tubes in correct order.
_____ 21. Mixes anticoagulated tubes promptly.
_____ 22. Fills tubes completely.
_____ 23. Removes last tube collected from holder.
_____ 24. Releases tourniquet within 1 minute.

_____ 25. Covers puncture site with gauze.
_____ 26. Removes the needle smoothly and applies pressure.
_____ 27. Activates needle safety device.
_____ 28. Disposes of the needle with safety device activated and attached to the holder in sharps container.
_____ 29. Labels tubes and confirms with the patient or ID band.
_____ 30. Examines puncture site.
_____ 31. Applies bandage.
_____ 32. Disposes of used supplies.
_____ 33. Removes gloves and washes hands.
_____ 34. Thanks patient.
_____ 35. Converses appropriately with patient during procedure.

Total points
Maximum points = 70
COMMENTS

REVIEW QUESTIONS

1. The most important step in the venipuncture procedure is:
   a. Applying the tourniquet
   b. Locating the best vein
   c. Identifying the patient
   d. Applying pressure to the puncture site

2. The minimum required number of patient identifiers required by the Joint Commission is:
   a. 1
   b. 2
   c. 3
   d. 4

3. To avoid interference with test results, the maximum time that a tourniquet can remain on the patient's arm is:
   a. 1 minute
   b. 2 minutes
   c. 5 minutes
   d. 10 minutes

4. The venipuncture step of primary importance to prevent rolling veins is:
   a. Tightly applying the tourniquet
   b. Selecting the median cubital vein
   c. Using a 23-gauge needle
   d. Anchoring the vein while inserting the needle

5. Areas from which blood should NOT be collected include all of the following EXCEPT:
   a. The basilic vein
   b. From a hematoma
   c. An arm with an IV running
   d. An arm with a fistula

6. The needle is inserted into the vein:
   a. Bevel up at a 45–50 degree angle
   b. Bevel up at a 15–30 degree angle
   c. Bevel down at a 15–30 degree angle
   d. Bevel down at a 45–50 degree angle

7. Bracing the hand holding the needle assembly against the patient's arm:
   a. Decreases the patient's discomfort
   b. Prevents excess needle movement
   c. Decreases the possibility of hemolysis
   d. Allows the tubes to fill more quickly

8. All of the following may cause hematoma formation EXCEPT:
   a. Removing the tourniquet after removing the needle
   b. Bandaging the patient's arm immediately after needle removal
   c. Firmly anchoring the vein in needle insertion
   d. Having the patient bend the elbow and apply pressure

9. Prior to bandaging the puncture site, the phlebotomist should:
   a. Thank the patient
   b. Instruct a fasting patient to eat
   c. Examine the site for bleeding
   d. Apply pressure for at least 5 minutes

10. Which of the following is performed first when the last tube is filled?
    a. Filled tube is removed from the holder
    b. Needle is withdrawn from the arm
    c. Gauze is placed over the needle
    d. Pressure is applied to the site

Internet Help

www.clsi.org
www.jcaho.org

www.bd.com/vacutainer/
labnotes

Complications and Additional Techniques

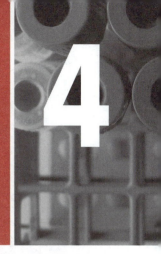

4

LEARNING OBJECTIVES

Upon completion of this unit, the reader will be able to:

- List the reasons why blood may not be immediately obtained from a venipuncture and the procedures to follow to obtain blood.
- List six causes of hematomas.
- Discuss the venipuncture errors that may produce hemolysis.
- Explain five causes of specimen contamination.
- Describe technical complications related to blood collection and the remedies for each situation.
- Discuss patient complications and an effective method to handle each situation.

- Identify the specific requirements related to blood collection in the elderly and pediatric populations.
- Describe the venipuncture procedure using a syringe, including equipment examination, technique for exchanging syringes, transfer of blood to evacuated tubes, and disposal of the equipment.
- Describe the venipuncture procedure using a winged blood collection set (butterfly), including technique involved and disposal of the equipment.
- List five reasons for rejecting a specimen.

Introduction

Patient and procedural complications can occur with blood collection. Technical complications with the venipuncture procedure result in the inability to obtain blood, a rejected specimen, or discomfort to the patient. This unit identifies the complications that can be encountered and remedies for each. Additional techniques for obtaining blood in these special situations are also emphasized.

Failure to Obtain Blood

The primary complication for the blood collector is the failure to obtain blood when the needle is inserted. **Figure 4–1** illustrates possible causes of failure to obtain blood. Slightly moving or turning the needle may result in blood flow without having to repuncture the patient.

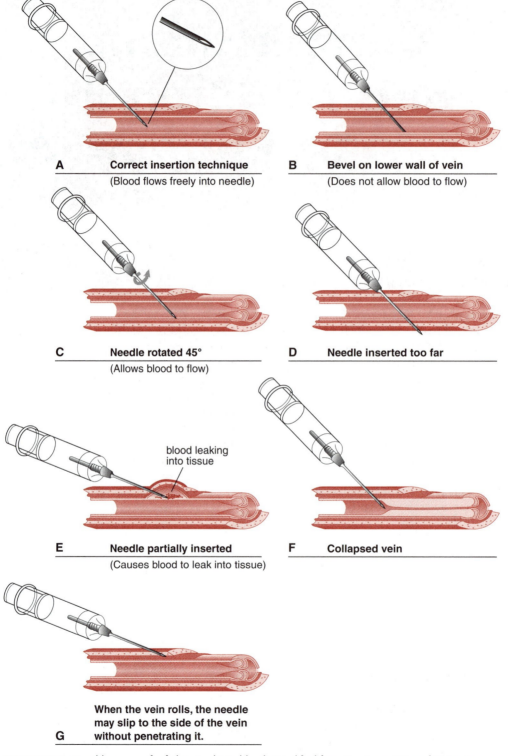

A   **Correct insertion technique**
(Blood flows freely into needle)

B   **Bevel on lower wall of vein**
(Does not allow blood to flow)

C   **Needle rotated 45°**
(Allows blood to flow)

D   **Needle inserted too far**

blood leaking
into tissue

E   **Needle partially inserted**
(Causes blood to leak into tissue)

F   **Collapsed vein**

G   **When the vein rolls, the needle
may slip to the side of the vein
without penetrating it.**

FIGURE 4–1. Possible reasons for failure to obtain blood. *(Modified from Strasinger, SK, and Di Lorenzo, MS: Phlebotomy Workbook, ed. 2. FA Davis, Philadelphia, 2003, Figure 7–5, p. 147, with permission.)*

A frequent reason for the failure to obtain blood occurs when a vein is not well anchored prior to the puncture. The needle may slip to the side of the vein without actual penetration ("rolling vein") (see Fig 4-1*G*). Gently touching the area around the needle with a cleansed gloved finger may determine the positions of the vein and the needle, and allow the needle to be slightly redirected. To avoid having to repuncture the patient, withdraw the needle until the bevel is just under the skin, reanchor the vein, and redirect the needle into the vein.

Blood flow may not occur when the angle of needle insertion is too steep (greater than 30 degrees) or when the tube holder is not kept steady when tubes are advanced onto the needle. The needle may penetrate through the vein into the tissue. Gently pulling the needle back may produce blood flow (see Fig. 4–1*D*).

If the needle angle is too shallow (less than 15 degrees), the needle may only partially enter the lumen of the vein, causing blood to leak into the tissues. Slowly advancing the needle into the vein may correct the problem (see Fig. 4–1*E*).

Blood flow also may be prevented when the bevel of the needle is resting against the upper or lower wall of the vein. Rotating the needle a quarter of a turn or pulling slightly back on the needle will allow blood to flow freely (see Figs. 4–1*B* and *C*).

If the needle appears to be in the vein, a faulty evacuated tube (either by manufacturer error, age of the tube, dropping the tube, or accidental puncture when assembling the equipment) may be the problem, and a new tube should be used. Remember to always have extra tubes within reach.

Using too large an evacuated tube or pulling back on the plunger of a syringe too quickly creates suction pressure that can cause a vein to collapse and stop blood flow (see Fig. 4–1*F*). Using a smaller evacuated tube or pulling more slowly on the syringe plunger may remedy the situation. If this does not help, another puncture must be performed, possibly using a syringe or a butterfly.

It is important for blood collectors to know these techniques to avoid having the patient unnecessarily repunctured.

Movement of the needle should not include blind or vigorous probing, because not only is this painful to the patient, but this also enlarges the puncture site and blood may leak into the tissues and form a hematoma. The most critical permanent injury in the venipuncture procedure that can be caused by vigorous probing is damage to the median antebrachial cutaneous nerve. Errors in technique that cause injury include selecting high-risk venipuncture sites, employing an excessive angle of needle insertion, and excessive manipulation of the needle. The Clinical and Laboratory Standards Institute (CLSI) standard H3-A6 limits needle redirection to only a forward or backward movement in a straight line. Lateral needle relocation of the needle to access the basilic vein is forbidden.

> **TECHNICAL TIP**
> According to the CLSI standard H3-A6, the needle should be inserted at an angle of less than 30 degrees.

When blood is not obtained from the initial venipuncture, the blood collector should select another site, either in the other arm or below the previous site, **and repeat the procedure using a new needle.** If the second puncture is not successful, the same person should not make another attempt. Possibly a phlebotomist from the clinical laboratory should attempt to collect the specimen.

Hematomas

Hematomas are caused by the leakage of blood into the tissues around the venipuncture site. The skin discoloration and swelling that accompanies a hematoma is often a cause of anxiety and discomfort to the patient, and can cause disabling compression injury to nerves. Improper technique when removing the needle is a frequent cause of the appearance of a hematoma on the patient's arm. Errors in technique that cause blood to leak or to be forced into the surrounding tissue and produce hematomas include the following:

1. Failing to remove the tourniquet prior to removing the needle
2. Applying inadequate pressure to the site after removal of the needle
3. Excessive probing to obtain blood
4. Failing to insert the needle far enough into the vein
5. Inserting the needle through the vein
6. Bending the arm while applying pressure
7. Using veins that are fragile or too small for the needle size

Under normal conditions, the elasticity of the vein walls prevents the leakage of blood around the needle during venipuncture. A decrease in the elasticity of the vein walls in older patients causes them to be more prone to developing hematomas. If the area begins to form a hematoma while blood is being collected, immediately remove the tourniquet and needle and apply pressure to the site for 2 minutes. Using small-bore needles and firmly anchoring the veins prior to needle insertion may prevent hematoma formation in these patients. A cold compress may be offered to the patient to minimize hematoma swelling and pain. Follow institutional policy.

The compromised venipuncture site is unacceptable for blood collection until the hematoma is resolved. An alternate site should be chosen for venipuncture, or if none is available, the venipuncture must be performed below the hematoma. The goal of successful blood collection is not only to obtain the sample, but also to preserve the site for future venipunctures. It is critical to prevent hematoma formation.

> **TECHNICAL TIP**
> Specimens collected following vigorous probing are frequently hemolyzed and must be recollected.

Nerve Injury

Temporary or permanent nerve damage can be caused by incorrect vein site selection or improper venipuncture technique and may result in loss of movement to the arm or hand, and the possibility of a lawsuit. Symptoms of nerve involvement are tingling, a burning or electric shock sensation, pain that is felt up and down the arm, or a numbness of the arm. The factors associated with nerve injury in blood collection are preventable and include:

- Improper vein selection
- Using jerky movements
- Inserting the needle too far
- Movement by the patient while the needle is in the vein
- Lateral redirection of the needle
- Blind probing

Hemolyzed Specimens

Hemolysis is detected by the presence of pink or red plasma or serum (**Fig. 4–2**). Rupture of the red blood cell membrane releases cellular contents into the serum or plasma that produces interference with many test results, which may require the specimen to be redrawn. **Table 4–1** summarizes the major tests affected by hemolysis.

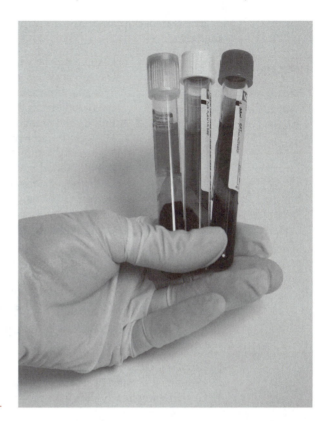

FIGURE 4-2. Slight, moderate, and gross serum hemolysis.

TABLE 4-1. Laboratory Tests Affected by Hemolysis

SERIOUSLY AFFECTED	NOTICEABLY AFFECTED	SLIGHTLY AFFECTED
Potassium (K)	Serum iron (Fe)	Phosphorus (P)
Lactic dehydrogenase (LD)	Alanine aminotransferase (ALT)	Total protein (TP)
Aspartate aminotransferase (AST)	Thyroxine (T4)	Albumin
Complete blood count (CBC)		Magnesium (Mg)
		Calcium (Ca)
		Acid phosphatase

Errors in performance of the venipuncture account for the majority of hemolyzed specimens and include:

1. Using a needle with too small a diameter (above 23-gauge)
2. Using a small needle with a large evacuated tube
3. Using an improperly attached needle on a syringe so that frothing occurs as the blood enters the syringe
4. Pulling the plunger of a syringe back too fast
5. Drawing blood from a site containing a hematoma
6. Vigorously mixing tubes
7. Forcing blood from a syringe into an evacuated tube
8. Collecting specimens from IV lines when not recommended by the manufacturer
9. Applying the tourniquet too close to the puncture site or for too long
10. Using fragile hand veins
11. Performing venipuncture before the alcohol is allowed to dry
12. Collecting blood through different internal diameters of catheters and connectors
13. Partially filling sodium fluoride tubes
14. Readjusting the needle in the vein or using occluded veins

Factors in processing, handling, or transporting the specimen can result in hemolyzed specimens and include:

1. Rimming clots
2. Prolonged contact of serum or plasma with cells
3. Centrifuging at a higher than recommended speed and with increased heat exposure in the centrifuge
4. Elevated or decreased temperatures of blood
5. Using pneumatic tube systems without shock-absorbing inserts padding the canister

Various patient physiological factors affect hemolysis and include metabolic disorders (liver disease, sickle cell anemia, autoimmune hemolytic anemia), chemical agents (lead, sulfonamides, antimalarial drugs, analgesics), physical agents (mechanical heart valve, third-degree burns), and infectious agents (parasites, bacteria).

Specimen Contamination

Specimen contamination affects the integrity of the specimen, causing invalid test results. The laboratory personnel may not know that contamination has occurred and consequently can report erroneous test results that adversely affect overall patient care. Incorrect blood collection techniques that cause contamination include:

1. Blood collected from edematous areas
2. Blood collected from veins with hematomas
3. Blood collected from arms containing an IV
4. Sites contaminated with alcohol or iodine
5. Anticoagulant carryover between tubes

Technical Problems

Rarely, the blood collector may encounter an evacuated tube that pops back or off of the tube stoppering needle while blood is being collected. Readvancing the tube onto the needle in the holder and holding it in this position until the tube is filled will remedy this situation. When using the evacuated tube system, always screw the needle onto the holder tightly. Needles have become unscrewed from the holder during venipuncture. If this happens, release the tourniquet immediately, and carefully remove the needle. Activate the safety device over the needle.

Reflux of a tube anticoagulant can occur when there is blood backflow into a patient's vein from the collection tube. This can cause adverse reactions in patients. Keeping the patient's arm and the tube in a downward position, allowing the collection tubes to fill from the bottom up, eliminates this problem.

Partially filled collection tubes deliver the wrong ratio of blood to anticoagulant, resulting in an inadequate specimen for laboratory testing. Light blue stopper tubes are the most affected because they contain liquid anticoagulant and the incorrect anticoagulant to blood ratio dilutes the plasma and causes erroneously prolonged coagulation results. The lavender stopper tube must be filled to avoid excess ethylenediaminetetraacetic acid (EDTA) shrinking the red blood cells and affecting the hematocrit, red blood cell count, hemoglobin, red blood cell indices, and erythrocyte sedimentation rate (ESR) results. ESRs must be analyzed within 4 hours of the specimen collection. Completely filled green stopper tubes are critical for ionized calcium tests. Underfilled gray stopper tubes cause hemolysis of the red blood cells. Serum separator tubes (SSTs) and red stopper tubes are usually not affected if there is an adequate amount of specimen to perform the test. "Partial draw" tubes are available for situations when it is difficult to obtain a full tube. These tubes have a smaller vacuum and a line on the tube indicates the proper fill level.

TECHNICAL TIP

To ensure prevention of reflux, blood in the tubes should not come in contact with the stopper during collection.

Patient Complications

Apprehensive patients may be prone to fainting (syncope). It is sometimes possible to detect such patients during vein palpation, because their skin may feel cold and damp. Other signs include pallor, perspiration, or the patient indicating that he or she feels light-headed, dizzy, or nauseous. The blood collector should ask the patient if he or she has had problems with blood collection or a tendency to faint. Having the patient lie down or using a blood collection chair with a locked armrest will prevent the patient from falling and injuring himself or herself. Keeping the patient's mind off the procedure through conversation may be helpful. If a patient begins to faint during the procedure, remove the tourniquet and needle and apply pressure to the venipuncture site. Make certain a patient who is not in bed is supported and that the patient lowers his or her head. Applying cold compresses to the forehead and back of the neck helps revive the patient. Outpatients who have been fasting for prolonged periods should be given something sweet to drink and be required to remain in the area for 15 to 30 minutes. All incidents of syncope should be documented according to institutional policy. According to the CLSI standard H3-A6, the use of ammonia inhalants for a fainting patient is not advised.

It is rare for patients to develop seizures during venipuncture. If this happens, the needle and tourniquet should be removed, pressure applied to the site, and help summoned. Restrain the

TECHNICAL TIP

Patients frequently mention previous adverse reactions. If these patients are sitting up, it may be wise to have them lie down prior to collection. It is not uncommon for patients with a history of fainting to faint again.

patient only to the extent that injury is prevented. Do not attempt to place anything in the patient's mouth. Any very deep puncture caused by sudden movement by the patient should be reported to the physician. Document the time the seizure started and stopped according to institutional policy.

Patients who present with small, nonraised red hemorrhagic spots (called petechiae) may have prolonged bleeding following venipuncture. Petechiae can be an indication of a coagulation disorder, such as a low platelet count or abnormal platelet function.

Patient medications may interfere with the clinical interpretation of some test results. Acetaminophen (Tylenol) and erythromycin can increase serum aspartate aminotransferase (AST) and bilirubin levels. Intravenous injections of medications and dyes also can interfere with laboratory analysis. Blood creatinine, cortisol, and digoxin levels can be altered by the intravenous fluorescein used in angiography procedures. If the blood collector is aware of a recent dye injection or patient medication, it should be noted on the requisition.

Medications that are toxic to the liver can cause an increase in blood liver enzymes and abnormal coagulation tests. Elevated blood urea nitrogen (BUN) levels or imbalanced electrolytes may be seen in patients taking medications that impair renal function. Patients taking corticosteroids, estrogens, or diuretics can develop pancreatitis and will have elevated serum amylase and lipase levels. Hypobilirubinemia can be caused by a patient taking aspirin, because bilirubin is expelled from the plasma to the surrounding tissue cells. Communication between the blood collector and the laboratory staff concerning possible interfering medications will ensure quality patient test results.

Special Patient Populations

Geriatric Population

Unique preparation and sometimes modifications to the blood collection technique are necessary to successfully accommodate the collection of blood from the pediatric and geriatric population. Blood collection in the older patient population presents a challenge to the blood collector. Physical, emotional, and physiological factors related to the aging process can cause difficulty with the blood collection procedure and specimen integrity. The goal is to perform a nontraumatic venipuncture without bruising or excessive bleeding and provide a quality specimen for analysis.

Normal aging often results in physical changes such as hearing loss; failing eyesight; loss of taste, smell, and feeling; and memory impairment. The blood collector must face the patient and speak clearly and repeat instructions if necessary. The patient may have to be guided to the blood drawing chair and have help being seated. Muscle weakness may cause the patient to be unable to make a fist before venipuncture or to hold the gauze after the venipuncture. Memory loss may cause the older patient to not remember medications he or she may have taken that can affect laboratory test results. A patient's inability to remember when he or she has last eaten can affect a test requiring fasting. Malnutrition or dehydration because of not eating or drinking adequately can make locating veins for venipuncture difficult because of decreased plasma volume and can affect laboratory results, by raising potassium levels.

Certain disease states such as Alzheimer disease, stroke, arthritis, coagulation disorders, and Parkinson disease affect the elderly and present challenges to blood collection. A patient with Alzheimer disease may be confused or combative, which can cause problems with identification and performing the procedure. Assistance from a family member or the patient's caretaker is often necessary to calm the patient and hold the arm steady. Stroke patients may have paralysis or speech impairments that require assistance in positioning and holding the arm and help with communication. Arthritic patients may be in pain or unable to straighten the arm and may require assistance gently positioning and holding the arm. Using a winged blood collection set with flexible tubing will allow the blood collector to access veins at awkward angles. Older patients are often on anticoagulant therapy for heart problems or stroke. Extra time is necessary to hold pressure on the site until bleeding has stopped before bandaging the area to avoid excessive bleeding or hematoma formation. Older patients may have tremors, as evidenced in Parkinson disease, and cannot hold the arm still for the venipuncture procedure. Patients often are embarrassed by these conditions, which may cause anxiety or fear of blood collection.

Physiologic changes in the aging process affect venipuncture. Epidermal cell replacement in the aging patient is delayed, increasing the chance of infection. If the patient already has a weakened immune system, the patient may not heal as quickly or have the ability to fight bacteria that can be introduced during venipuncture. Extra care must be taken when preparing the site for venipuncture. With aging, the loss of collagen and subcutaneous tissue makes the veins less elastic and fragile with a tendency to collapse. The veins are harder to anchor and puncture and more prone to hematoma formation. The blood collector must firmly anchor the vein below the site so that the vein does not move when it is punctured. Loose skin can be pulled taut by wrapping your hand around the arm from behind. The angle of the needle may need to be decreased for venipuncture because the veins are often close to the surface. Arteries and veins often become sclerotic in the older patient, making them poor sites for venipuncture because of the compromised blood flow.

The difficulty in locating and anchoring veins and the presence of hematomas from previous venipunctures in the elderly patient often result in the antecubital fossa to not be the best site selection. The veins in the hand or forearm may be a better choice. It may require taking a little extra time and using the techniques previously described for making veins more prominent. Warming the site can make the vein more prominent but never tap the vein to avoid bruising the patient.

EQUIPMENT SELECTION

The evacuated tube system is usually not the best choice for venipuncture on the elderly because the vacuum pressure in the collection tube may cause fragile veins to collapse. A better choice is a butterfly needle (winged blood collection set) with a 23-gauge needle attached to a syringe that will allow the blood collector to control the suction pressure on the vein. A small gauge needle with a syringe is also an option. Pediatric or partial-draw tubes should be used because of the tendency to develop anemia by older patients; therefore, the volume of blood collected should be kept to the minimum acceptable amount. Blood pressure cuffs can be used for the thin patient with small, hard-to-find veins. Elderly patients are prone to bruising when applying the tourniquet or adhesive bandages. The tourniquet can be placed over the patient's sleeve and must not be applied too tightly to avoid injury. It is preferable to use a self-adhering bandage because adhesive bandages on the fragile skin of older patients can actually take off a layer of skin when they are removed and leave a raw wound susceptible to infection. A better alternative is for the blood collector to hold pressure on the site for 3 to 5 minutes or until the bleeding has stopped.

Dermal puncture, when possible, should be performed on the older patient as a way of avoiding complications, such as hematomas, bruising, collapsed veins, and anemia. The advances in point-of-care testing have made it possible to perform many types of tests on a small amount of blood that can be obtained by dermal puncture.

Pediatric Population

Ideally, children younger than 2 years of age should have blood collected by dermal puncture procedure. However, special tests for coagulation, erythrocyte sedimentation rates, special diagnostic studies, or blood cultures require more blood than can be collected from a finger or heel stick and must be collected by venipuncture. Pediatric blood collection involves preparing both the child and parent, using certain restraining procedures, and special equipment. Pediatric phlebotomy presents emotional as well as technical difficulties and should be performed by only experienced blood collectors. It is important to keep the patient as calm as possible during the procedure because emotional stress and crying can affect blood analytes and cause erroneous test results. The minimum amount of blood should be collected for testing because infants and children have smaller blood volumes.

Assistance is usually required when collecting blood from a small child. Physical restraint may be required to immobilize the young child and steady the arm for the venipuncture procedure. This can be accomplished by having someone hold the child or by using a papoose board. Either a vertical or horizontal restraint will work. In the vertical position, the parent holds the child in an upright position on the lap. The parent places an arm around the toddler to hold the arm not being used. The other arm holds the child's venipuncture arm firmly from behind, at the bend of the elbow, in a downward position.

In the horizontal restraint, the child lies down, with the parent on one side of the bed and the blood collector on the opposite side. The parent leans over the child holding the near arm and body securely while reaching over the body to hold the opposite venipuncture arm for the blood collector.

EQUIPMENT SELECTION

The minimum amount of blood required for laboratory testing should be collected from infants and small children because drawing excessive amounts of blood can cause anemia. The amount of blood collected within a 24-hour period must be monitored because of the small blood volume in newborns and small children. When using an evacuated tube system, select the smallest evacuated pediatric tubes available to collect the least amount of blood and to avoid causing the vein to collapse. Evacuated tubes as small as 1.8 mL are available. A 23-gauge winged blood collection set needle with a syringe is recommended because of the small fragile veins. If only a very small amount of blood is collected, use a microcollection tube rather than an evacuated tube. Pediatric-sized tourniquets also are available.

A local topical anesthetic, eutectic mixture of local anesthetics (EMLA) is ideal for use on an apprehensive child before venipuncture. This emulsion of lidocaine and prilocaine is applied directly to intact skin and covered with an occlusive dressing. EMLA penetrates to a depth of 5 mm through the epidermal and dermal layer of the skin. It takes 60 minutes to reach its optimum effect and lasts for 2 or 3 hours. EMLA should not be used on infants younger than 1 month of age or if the child is allergic to local anesthetics. One side effect of this emulsion may be pallor at the site or a slight redness because of the adhesive covering.

It has been shown that a sucrose solution has a calming effect on infants. Commercial sucrose pacifiers or nipples are available. A 24-percent solution of sucrose may be made by mixing 4 teaspoons of water with 1 teaspoon of sugar. This sucrose solution may be given to the infant using a syringe, dropper, nipple, or pacifier about 2 minutes before venipuncture, and the effects last for about 5 minutes.

SITE SELECTION

The veins located in the antecubital fossa or the forearm are the best choice for children older than 2 years of age. Do not use deep veins. Dorsal hand veins are preferred sites for infants.

Use of Syringes

Except for a few minor differences, the procedure for drawing blood using a syringe is the same as when using an evacuated tube system. Blood is withdrawn from the vein by slowly pulling on the plunger of the syringe using the hand that is free after the anchored vein is entered. The advantage of using a syringe is that when the vein is entered, blood will appear in the hub of the needle and the plunger can then be pulled back at a speed that corresponds to the rate of blood flow into the syringe. Pulling the plunger back faster than the rate of blood flow may cause the walls of the vein to collapse (**see Fig. 4–1F**) and can cause hemolysis. Pulling the plunger back too slowly may cause the blood to begin to clot in the syringe before the blood is collected and transferred to anticoagulated tubes. It is important to anchor the hand holding the syringe firmly on the patient's arm so that the needle will not move when the plunger is pulled.

Ideally, the size of the syringe used should correspond to the amount of blood needed. It may be necessary to fill two or more smaller syringes when veins are small and may easily collapse. This will require assistance, because blood from the filled syringe must be transferred to the appropriate tubes while the second syringe is being filled. It is important that blood be added to anticoagulated tubes as soon as possible. Before exchanging syringes, gauze must be placed on the patient's arm under the needle because blood will leak from the hub of the needle during the exchange.

As discussed in Unit 2, blood is transferred from the syringe to evacuated tubes, following the prescribed order of fill, using a blood transfer device. After removing the needle from the vein, activate the needle safety device and remove the needle and discard it in the sharps container. The blood transfer device is attached to the syringe and evacuated tubes are pushed onto the stopper-puncturing rubber-sheathed needle. After the tubes are filled, the syringe and blood transfer device are discarded into a sharps container. The venipuncture procedure using a syringe is shown in **Figure 4–3.**

TECHNICAL TIP

In most circumstances, the use of small evacuated tubes with a winged blood collection set instead of a syringe can prevent the need to change syringes.

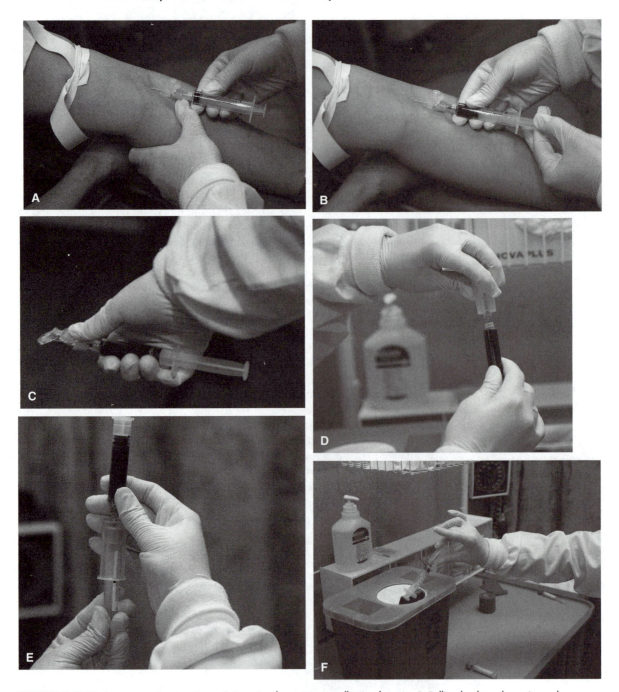

FIGURE 4–3. Venipuncture using a syringe. *A,* Inserting the syringe needle into the vein. *B,* Pulling back on the syringe plunger. *C,* Removing the needle from the vein and activating the safety device. *D,* Attaching the blood transfer device to the syringe. *E,* Advancing the tube onto the internal needle in the blood transfer device. *F,* Syringe assembly disposal.

Use of Winged Blood Collection Sets

All routine venipuncture procedures used with evacuated tubes and syringes also apply to blood collection using a winged blood collection set (butterfly). This method is used for difficult venipuncture and is often less painful to patients. The angle of needle insertion can be lowered to 10 to 15 degrees facilitating entry into small veins by folding the plastic needle attachments ("wings") upward while inserting the needle. Blood will appear in the tubing when the vein is entered. The needle can then be threaded securely into the vein and kept in place by holding the plastic wings against the patient's arm. It may be helpful to have a piece of tape available in case two hands are needed for the collection. Depending on the type of winged blood collection set used, blood can be collected into an evacuated tube or a syringe. The tubing contains a small amount of air that will cause underfilling of the first tube; therefore, a discard tube should be collected before a coagulation tube to maintain the correct blood to anticoagulant ratio. To prevent hemolysis when using a small (23-gauge) needle, small volume evacuated tubes should be used. When using a winged blood collection set, be sure to attach the holder to the stopper-puncturing needle and not just push the tubes onto the back of the rubber sheathed needle. This will avoid an accidental needlestick exposure from the stopper-puncturing needle. Tubes are positioned downward to fill from the bottom up and in the same order of draw as in evacuated tube venipuncture. If blood has been collected into a syringe, the winged blood collection needle safety device is activated and removed from the syringe. A blood transfer device is attached to the syringe (**see Fig. 4–3F**) and the evacuated tubes are filled in the correct order.

SAFETY TIP
Always hold a butterfly apparatus by the wings, not by the tubing.

When disposing of the winged blood collection set, use extreme care, because many accidental sticks result from unexpected movement of the tubing. Immediately activating the needle safety device and placing the needle into a sharps container and then allowing the tubing to fall into the container when the evacuated tube or syringe is removed can prevent accidents. Using an apparatus with automatic resheathing capability or activating a device on the needle set that advances a safety blunt before removing the needle from the vein is recommended to prevent accidental needle punctures. Do not push the apparatus manually into a full sharps container.

The venipuncture procedure using a winged blood collection set is shown in **Figure 4–4**.

Causes of Specimen Rejection

Specimens brought to the laboratory may be rejected if conditions are present that would compromise the validity of the test results.

Major reasons for specimen rejection are the following:

1. Unlabeled or mislabeled specimens
2. Inadequate volume
3. Collection in the wrong tube
4. Hemolysis
5. Lipemia
6. Clotted blood in an anticoagulant tube
7. Improper handling during transport, such as not chilling the specimen
8. Specimens without a requisition form
9. Contaminated specimen containers
10. Delays in processing the specimen
11. Use of outdated blood collection tubes

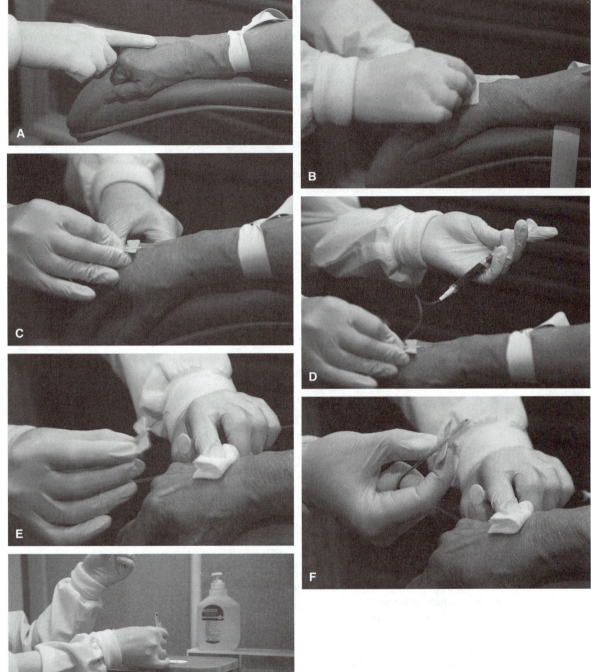

FIGURE 4–4. Venipuncture using a winged blood collection set. *A,* Hand vein palpation. *B,* Cleansing the puncture site. *C,* Inserting the needle. *D,* Collecting blood in a syringe. *E,* Removing the needle. *F,* Activating the needle safety device. *G,* Disposing of the winged blood collection set.

Venipuncture Complication Situations Exercise

1. An unidentified patient in the emergency room requires a transfusion. What precautions must the blood collector take?

   _____

   _____

   _____

2. The blood collector has a requisition to collect blood for a metabolic profile and a pro-thrombin time (PT). No blood is obtained from the left antecubital area. The blood collector then moves to the right antecubital area and obtains a full gold stopper tube, but cannot fill the light blue stopper tube. What should the blood collector do next?

   _____

   _____

   _____

3. A patient has an IV drip running in the left forearm. From the following sites, indicate your first choice with a "1," your second choice with a "2," and an unacceptable site with an "X."

   a. _____ left wrist

   b. _____ left antecubital area

   c. _____ right antecubital area

4. The blood collector with a requisition for a PT, complete blood count (CBC), and rheumatoid arthritis (RA) on a patient who is difficult to draw obtains 7 mL of blood using a syringe. Assuming the blood collector has a 2.7-mL light blue stopper tube, a 2-mL lavender stopper tube, and a 3-mL red stopper tube, how should the blood be distributed?

   _____

   _____

   _____

5. A blood collector needs to collect 20 mL of blood for serum chemistry tests and selects two 10-mL SST tubes. A successful puncture is performed; however, blood stops flowing when the first tube is only half full.

   a. Assuming the problem is not with the equipment, what is a possible reason for this?

   _____

   _____

   _____

   b. State two methods the blood collector could use to collect the required amount of blood.

   _____

   _____

   _____

6. When collecting a specimen from an elderly patient using routine evacuated tube equipment, the blood collector notices that the puncture site is beginning to swell.

   a. Why is this happening?

   _____

   b. What should the blood collector do?

   _____

   c. How can the specimen be collected?

   _____

7. While blood for a CBC is being collected, the patient develops syncope and the blood collector removes the needle and lowers the patient's head. Once the patient has recovered, the blood collector labels the lavender stopper tube, which contains enough blood, and delivers it to the clinical laboratory. Many results from this specimen are markedly lower than those from the patient's previous CBC.

   a. How could the quality of the specimen have caused this discrepancy?

   _____

   _____

   b. How could the venipuncture complication have contributed to this error?

   _____

   _____

   c. Could the blood collector have done anything differently? Explain your answer.

   _____

   _____

8. Patients in the cardiac care unit are exhibiting an unusual number of hematomas. Considering the condition and treatment of the patients in this unit, what is the most probable error being made by the blood collectors? Explain your answer.

   _____

   _____

   _____

9. The blood collector sends a properly labeled specimen with sufficient volume collected in a light green stopper tube to the clinical laboratory for a potassium determination. Fifteen minutes later the chemistry supervisor calls and asks that the specimen be redrawn.

   a. Why did the chemistry supervisor reject this specimen?

   _____

   b. What precautions should the blood collector take with the second specimen?

   _____

   _____

   _____

10. An elderly patient who recently had open-heart surgery regularly comes to the physician's office laboratory for her PT test to monitor her Coumadin therapy.

a. What precautions must be taken when applying tourniquet and adhesive bandages?

_____

_____

_____

b. State the preferable venipuncture equipment used for geriatric patients?

_____

_____

_____

c. What error in technique can cause a compromised PT test result?

_____

_____

_____

d. Name four complications in performing venipuncture on the geriatric patient.

_____

_____

_____

e. What extra precautions must be taken before bandaging the patient?

_____

_____

_____

11. An extremely overweight man came to the physician's office laboratory with a requisition for a metabolic profile. The blood collector had a difficult time finding a good median cubital or cephalic vein; however, she did feel a deep basilic vein. Inserting the needle at a greater than 30-degree angle and after much probing, the blood collector was able to obtain the blood. The patient complained of a burning, tingling sensation up and down his arm.

a. What caused the tingling sensation?

_____

_____

_____

b. What is the CLSI recommendation needle angle and vein selection?

_____

_____

_____

c. What other complication may have occurred that would cause the lab to reject the specimen?

_____

_____

_____

REVIEW QUESTIONS

1. When blood is not obtained when the needle is inserted all of the following techniques may be tried EXCEPT:
   a. Gently advancing the needle
   b. Gently pulling the needle back
   c. Redirecting the needle to the side
   d. Inserting a new tube into the holder

2. Which of the following is most critically affected in a hemolyzed specimen?
   a. Potassium
   b. Albumin
   c. Total protein
   d. Calcium

3. The first thing the collector should do when a patient develops syncope is:
   a. Lower the patient's head
   b. Apply cold compresses to the patient's neck
   c. Remove the tourniquet and needle
   d. Place the patient on a bed

4. When blood collected in a syringe must be placed in evacuated tubes:
   a. The needle safety device is activated
   b. The needle is discarded
   c. A blood transfer device is attached to the syringe
   d. All of the above

5. When performing venipuncture on a pediatric patient, the collector may require:
   a. Assistance
   b. A pediatric requisition
   c. Small evacuated tubes
   d. Both a and c

6. Older patients are more prone to hematoma formation because:
   a. They have smaller veins
   b. Tourniquets must be tied tighter
   c. Their veins have decreased elasticity
   d. They have difficulty making a fist

7. If the plunger of a syringe is pulled back too fast:
   a. The patients feel a stinging sensation
   b. The specimen may be hemolyzed
   c. The patient will develop a hematoma
   d. Both a and b

8. Specimens are rejected by the laboratory for all of the following reasons EXCEPT:
   a. Clots in a lavender stopper tube
   b. Collection in the wrong tube
   c. Incompletely filled light blue stopper tubes
   d. Clots in a red stopper tube

9. When an evacuated tube is pushed onto the needle, blood begins to flow and then stops. This could be caused by all of the following EXCEPT:
   a. Use of a 21-gauge needle
   b. Collapsing of the vein
   c. The bevel of the needle resting on the vein wall
   d. An occluded vein

10. The plastic wings on a winged blood collection set:
    a. Help hold the needle in place after insertion
    b. Allow the angle of insertion to be lowered
    c. Allow the angle of insertion to be raised
    d. Both a and b

Internet Help

www.clsi.org

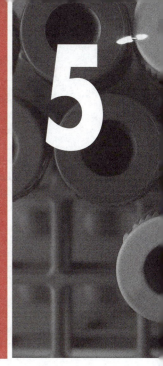

Special Venipuncture Collection and Preanalytical Variables

5

LEARNING OBJECTIVES

Upon completion of this unit, the reader will be able to:

- Explain the requirements for a 2-hour post-prandial glucose test and a glucose tolerance test (GTT).
- Discuss diurnal variation of blood constituents and list three substances that would be affected.
- Differentiate between a trough and a peak level in therapeutic drug monitoring.
- Discuss the timing sequences for the collection of blood cultures, the reasons for selecting a particular timing sequence, and the number of specimens collected.

- Describe the procedure for collecting specimens for cold agglutinins.
- List eight tests for which specimens must be chilled immediately after collection.
- List five tests for which the results are affected by exposure of the specimen to light.
- Define chain of custody.

Introduction

Certain laboratory tests require the use of techniques that are not part of the routine venipuncture procedure. These nonroutine procedures may involve patient preparation, timing of specimen collection, venipuncture techniques, and specimen handling. The blood collector must know when these techniques are required, how to perform them, and how specimen integrity is affected when they are not performed.

Fasting and Timed Specimens

Assessment of the patient preparation is necessary before blood collection for laboratory tests that require the patient to be fasting or in a basal state. It is the responsibility of the blood collector to verify that the patient has not had anything to eat or drink, except water, (fasting) and has refrained from strenuous exercise for 12 hours (basal state). Drinking water is encouraged to avoid dehydration in the patient, which can affect laboratory results. Specimens for fasting blood sugar (FBS), cholesterol, triglycerides, and cardiac risk profiles are the most critically affected by nonfasting. If the patient has not fasted, it must be noted on the requisition form. Prolonged fasting increases bilirubin and triglyceride results and markedly decreases glucose levels.

For GTTs, the fasting patient should be instructed to abstain from food and drinks, including coffee and unsweetened tea, except water for 12 hours but not more than 16 hours before and during the test. Smoking and chewing tobacco or sugarless gum should be avoided before and during the test because they stimulate digestion and may cause inaccurate test results. Note on the requisition form if the patient is chewing gum.

Blood collections are frequently requested for specific times, and the timing of specimen collection must be strictly followed for accurate test results. Reasons for timed specimens include measuring of the body's ability to metabolize a particular substance, monitoring changes in a patient's condition, determining blood levels of medications, measuring substances that exhibit diurnal variation, and measuring cardiac markers following an acute myocardial infarction. Collecting a specimen early could yield a falsely elevated result, whereas collecting the specimen late could yield a falsely normal result. Misinterpretation of test results can cause improper treatment for the patient. Frequently encountered timed specimens are the 2-hour postprandial glucose, GTT, therapeutic drug monitoring, anticoagulant therapy monitoring, and tests for substances that exhibit diurnal variation.

Two-Hour Postprandial Glucose

TECHNICAL TIP

A specimen that appears lipemic is an indication that the patient was not fasting and the lipemia may interfere with laboratory testing.

The 2-hour postprandial glucose test compares a patient's fasting glucose level with a glucose level 2 hours after eating a meal or ingesting a measured amount of glucose. It is used to screen for diabetes mellitus or gestational diabetes. Ideally, the glucose level should return to the fasting level within 2 hours.

Patients are instructed to be on a high-carbohydrate diet for 2 days before the test. The blood collector must confirm that the patient has ingested a meal equivalent to 100 g of glucose and collect the blood exactly 2 hours after the meal is ingested.

Glucose Tolerance Test

The GTT is a procedure performed for the diagnosis of diabetes mellitus (hyperglycemia) and for the evaluation of persons with symptoms associated with low blood glucose (hypoglycemia). The GTT may compare glucose results on blood and urine collected at appropriate times. The specimen collection schedule can range from a 1-hour test for gestational diabetes to a 3- or 6-hour test and is based on the time the patient finishes drinking the glucose solution. GTT procedures should be scheduled to begin between 0700 and 0900, because glucose levels exhibit a diurnal variation.

Patients are instructed to eat a balanced diet that includes 150 g per day of carbohydrates for 3 days and to fast for 12 hours before the test. Certain medications interfere with the test results (**Box 5–1**) and the patient should be instructed to tell the blood collector of any medication he or she is taking before beginning the test. A fasting glucose to determine whether the patient can

> ### BOX 5–1. Medications That May Interfere With GTT
>
> Alcohol
> Anticonvulsants
> Aspirin
> Birth control pills
> Blood pressure medications
> Corticosteroids
> Diuretics
> Estrogen-replacement pills

safely be given a large amount of glucose is collected and tested prior to beginning the procedure. The patient drinks a standardized amount of flavored glucose (Glucola) based on weight within 5 minutes (**Fig. 5–1**). Children and small adults receive 1 gram per kilogram of body weight. The timing for the collection of the GTT specimens begins when the patient finishes drinking the glucose. Sample schedules are shown in **Table 5–1**.

Outpatients are given a copy of the schedule and instructed to continue fasting, to drink water as needed, and to return to the drawing station at the scheduled times. Patients are usually instructed to remain in the outpatient area.

> **TECHNICAL TIP**
>
> Closely observe the patient for symptoms of hyperglycemia or hypoglycemia when collecting GTT specimens.

Labels containing routinely required information and specimen order in the test sequence, such as ½ hour, 1 hour, 2 hours, and so on, are placed on the specimens. Venous blood samples are preferred and the type of evacuated tube used must be consistent. Blood specimens that will not be tested until the end of the sequence should be collected in gray stopper tubes. Timing of specimen collection is critical, because test results are related to the scheduled times; any discrepancies should be noted on the requisition. Consistency of venipuncture

FIGURE 5–1. Glucose tolerance test beverage: 50-gram, 75-gram, and 100-gram doses.

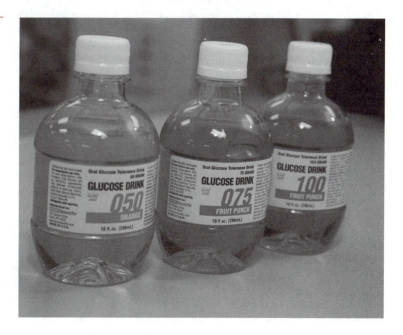

TABLE 5–1. Sample Glucose Tolerance Test Schedules		
TEST PROCEDURE	**3-HOUR TEST**	**6-HOUR TEST**
Fasting blood	0700	0700
Patient finishes glucose	0800	0800
½-hour specimen	0830	0830
1-hour specimen	0900	0900
2-hour specimen	1000	1000
3-hour specimen	1100	1100
4-hour specimen		1200
5-hour specimen		1300
6-hour specimen		1400

TECHNICAL TIP

Outpatients must understand the importance of adhering to the scheduled blood collection times for accurate results.

or dermal puncture also must be maintained, because glucose values differ between the two types of blood.

Some patients may not be able to tolerate the glucose solution, and if vomiting occurs, the time of the vomiting must be reported and the physician must be contacted for a decision concerning whether to continue the test. Vomiting early in the procedure is considered most critical and usually requires the procedure to be rescheduled.

Diurnal Variation

In addition to glucose, other substances such as cortisol, testosterone, estradiol, progesterone, renin, thyroid-stimulating hormone (TSH), serum iron, and white blood cells (most often eosinophils) also exhibit diurnal variation, and the levels of these substances fluctuate noticeably throughout the day. Certain variations can be substantial. For example, plasma cortisol levels collected between 0800 and 1000 will be twice as high as levels collected at 1600, and serum iron levels collected in the morning are one-third higher than those collected in the evening. Specimens must be collected at the specified time or the physician should be notified and the test rescheduled for the next day.

Therapeutic Drug Monitoring

The blood levels of some therapeutic drugs are monitored to ensure safety and medication effectiveness. Frequently monitored drugs include digoxin, procainamide, gentamicin, tobramycin, vancomycin, Dilantin, valproic acid, and theophylline. Random specimens are occasionally requested; however, the most beneficial levels are the trough and peak levels. The trough level is collected 30 minutes before the next dose of medication is scheduled and represents the lowest

TECHNICAL TIP

Depending on the half-life of the medication, the timing of peak levels in therapeutic drug monitoring can be critical.

level in the blood. Ideally, trough levels should be tested before administering the next dose to ensure that the level is low enough for the patient to receive more medication safely. The peak level is collected after medication administration at the time when the manufacturer specifies that the blood level should be at the highest point. The time of the peak level varies with the medication, the patient's metabolism, and the method of administration (intravenous, intramuscular, or oral). To ensure correct documentation of peak and trough levels, requisitions and specimen tube labels should include the time and method of administration of the last dose given, as well as the time that the specimen is collected. Therapeutic drug monitoring collections must be coordinated with the pharmacy, laboratory, and nursing staff.

Blood Cultures

Blood cultures are requested to detect septicemia in febrile patients. Specimens are usually collected in sets of two, drawn either 30 minutes to 1 hour apart or just before the patient's temperature spikes. If antibiotics are to be started immediately, the sets are drawn at the same time from different sites. Specimens collected from multiple sites at the same time serve as controls for possible contamination and must be labeled as to the collection site, such as right arm antecubital vein, and their number in the series (#1, #2). A known skin contaminant must be cultured from at least two of the sites for it to be considered a possible pathogen.

Blood for the culture may be drawn directly into bottles containing culture media, transferred to the bottles from a syringe, or drawn into sterile, yellow stopper evacuated tubes containing anticoagulant and transferred to culture media in the laboratory. Each set should be collected in the same manner as the first set. An anticoagulant must be present in the tube or the medium to prevent microorganisms from being trapped within a clot, where they might be undetected. Blood culture bottles must be mixed after the blood is added. The anticoagulant sodium polyanethol sulfonate (SPS) is used for blood cultures because it does not inhibit bacterial growth and may enhance it by inhibiting the action of phagocytes, complement, and some antibiotics. Other anticoagulants should not be used because bacterial growth may be inhibited. Some blood culture collection systems have antimicrobial removal devices (ARDs) containing a resin that inactivates antibiotics. **Figure 5–2** shows the equipment used in aseptic blood culture collection.

A winged blood collection set with a Luer adapter and a specially designed holder can be used to transfer blood directly from the patient to bottles containing culture media. The Luer adapter on the butterfly apparatus attaches

> ### SAFETY TIP
>
> Occupational Safety & Health Administration (OSHA) regulations require using a blood transfer device for transferring the blood. The earlier practice of putting a new needle on the syringe to inoculate the blood culture bottle directly is no longer acceptable.

FIGURE 5–2. Blood culture equipment.

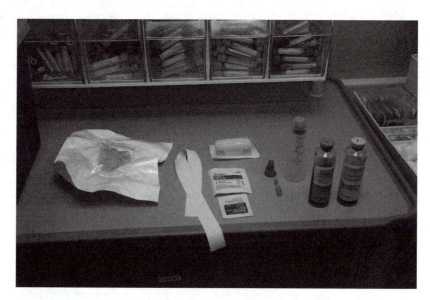

to the transfer device that contains a stopper-puncturing needle. Blood flows from the vein through the butterfly tubing, Luer adapter, and stopper-puncturing needle into the culture bottle. Fill the aerobic bottle first because the butterfly tubing has air in it. Do not allow the culture media to contact the stopper or needle during blood collection.

Blood can be collected in a syringe and aseptically transferred to blood culture bottles at the bedside, as shown in **Figure 5–3.** The anaerobic blood culture vial must be filled first.

Strict adherence to aseptic technique during specimen collection is essential to ensure that a positive blood culture is not caused by external contamination. Cleansing of the venipuncture site begins by vigorous scrubbing of the site with isopropyl alcohol for 60 seconds. The alcohol is followed by povidone-iodine or 2-percent iodine tincture applied by starting in the center of the site and progressing outward 3 to 4 inches in concentric circles. The iodine must be allowed to dry for 1 minute. To prevent irritation of the arm, remove the iodine with alcohol when the procedure is complete. Some health-care facilities are using chlorhexidine gluconate/isopropyl alcohol (ChloraPrep, Medi-Flex, Cardinal Health, Leawood, KS) because of the incidence of iodine sensitivity. It is a 30–60 second one-step vigorous scrub creating a friction (**Fig. 5–3A**). The site should not be repalpated after the venipuncture site has been sterilized; however, if the site must be touched after cleansing, the gloved palpating finger must be cleaned in the same manner. The tops of the collection containers are also cleaned before inoculating them with blood. The plastic caps are removed and the rubber stoppers can be cleaned using 70-percent alcohol only and covered with the alcohol pad until ready for inoculation or with iodine that is allowed to dry and then wiped off with alcohol (**Figs. 5–3B and C**). The iodine should not remain on the stoppers because it can enter the culture during specimen inoculation and may cause deterioration of some stoppers during incubation. Two specimens are routinely collected for each blood culture set, one to be incubated aerobically and the other to be incubated anaerobically. When a syringe is used, the anaerobic bottle should be inoculated first to prevent possible exposure to air. When the specimen is collected using a winged blood collection set, the aerobic bottle is inoculated first so that the air in the tubing does not enter the anaerobic bottle. As with all syringe-to-tube transfers, a transfer device is used. Do not inoculate directly from the syringe to the bottle (**Fig. 5–3G**).

A 1:10 ratio of blood to culture medium is critical, because the number of microorganisms present in the blood is often small. Underfilled blood culture bottles may cause false-negative results. Overfilling of bottles should be avoided because this may cause false-positive results with automated systems. Read the bottle label for the size of blood sample required. Pediatric collection containers are available. Pediatric blood culture volume requirements are based on the child's weight. Draw 1 mL of blood from babies weighing less than 5 kg, and place all the blood in one pediatric bottle.

> **TECHNICAL TIP**
>
> Wearing sterile gloves is recommended for aseptic technique in the collection of blood cultures.

> **TECHNICAL TIP**
>
> The Clinical and Laboratory Standards Institute (CLSI) recommends removing the dried alcohol or iodine from the blood culture stopper with clean gauze prior to inoculation.

Special Specimen Handling Procedures

Instructions for the collection, transportation, and storage of all laboratory specimens are available from the laboratory and should be strictly followed to maintain specimen integrity. Some tests require that the specimen be kept warm, chilled, frozen, or protected from light.

Cold Agglutinins

Cold agglutinins are autoantibodies produced by persons infected with *Mycoplasma pneumoniae*. The autoantibodies react with red blood cells (RBCs) at temperatures below body temperature. Because the cold agglutinins in the serum attach to RBCs when the blood cools to

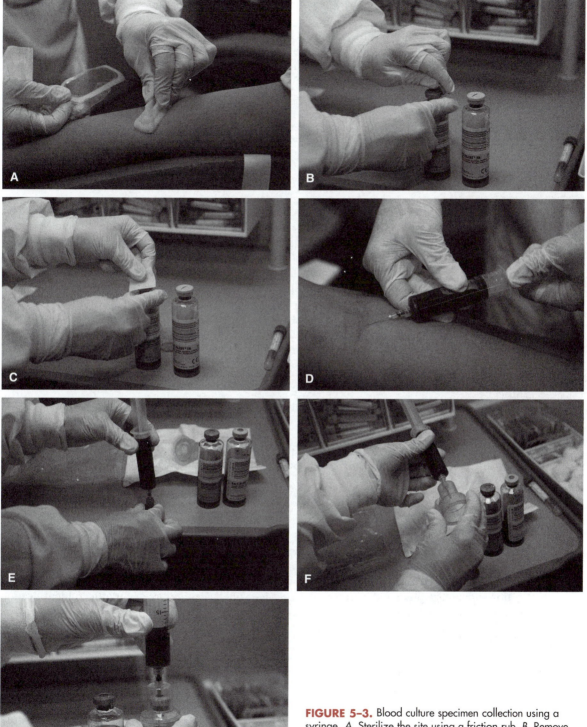

FIGURE 5-3. Blood culture specimen collection using a syringe. *A*, Sterilize the site using a friction rub. *B*, Remove plastic cap on collection bottle. *C*, Clean and cover tops of bottles with 70% isopropyl alcohol pad. *D*, Perform the venipuncture. *E*, Remove syringe needle with a Point-Lok device. *F*, Attach transfer device. *G*, Inoculate blood culture bottles.

below body temperature, the specimen must be kept warm until the serum can be separated from the cells. Specimens are collected in tubes that have been warmed in an incubator at 37°C for 30 minutes and that contain no additives or gels that could interfere with the test. The warmed tube is carried to the patient's room in the blood collector's tightly closed fist or a prewarmed container. The specimen is collected as quickly as possible and immediately delivered to the laboratory in the same manner. Failure to keep a specimen warm prior to serum separation produces falsely decreased test results. Cryofibrinogen and cryoglobulin are two proteins that precipitate when cold and must be collected and handled in the same manner as cold agglutinins.

TECHNICAL TIP

The CLSI recommends not to ice arterial blood gases (ABGs) when they have been collected in plastic syringes and analyzed within 30 minutes unless they are collected in conjunction with lactic acid.

Chilled Specimens

Specimens for arterial blood gases (if indicated), ammonia, acetone, free fatty acids, lactic acid, pyruvate, glucagons, gastrin, adrenocorticotropic hormone (ACTH), parathyroid hormone (PTH), renin, angiotensin-converting enzyme (ACE), catecholamines, homocysteine, and some coagulation studies must be chilled immediately after collection to prevent deterioration. For adequate chilling, the specimen must be placed in a mixture of crushed ice and water at the bedside or in a uniform ice block (**Fig. 5–4**). Placing a specimen in or on ice cubes is not acceptable, because uniform chilling will not occur. It is important that these specimens be immediately delivered to the laboratory for processing.

TECHNICAL TIP

Bilirubin is rapidly destroyed in specimens exposed to light and can decrease up to 50 percent after 1 hour of exposure to light.

Specimens Sensitive to Light

Exposure to light will decrease the concentration of bilirubin, beta-carotene, folate, vitamins A, B_{12}, and B_6, and porphyrins. Wrapping the tubes in aluminum foil or using an amber-colored transport bag can protect specimens (**Fig. 5–5**). Tubes should be kept closed. Refer to Unit 1 for proper preparation and transport of specimens from off-site collection facilities.

Legal Specimens

The chain of custody must be followed exactly when drawing specimens for test results that may be used as evidence in legal proceedings. Special forms are provided for the documentation of specimen handling, and special containers and seals may be required. Documentation must include the date, time, and identification of each person handling the specimen. Specimens should not be left sitting on a counter unattended. Patient identification and specimen collection should take place in the presence of a witness, often a law enforcement officer. Identification requires specific documents and may require photographs, fingerprints, or heel prints. The tests requested most frequently are alcohol and drug levels and DNA analysis.

TECHNICAL TIP

Technical errors and failure to follow chain of custody protocol are primary targets of the defense in legal proceedings.

When collecting blood alcohol levels, the site should be cleansed with soap and water or a nonalcoholic antiseptic solution, such as benzalkonium chloride. To prevent the escape of the volatile alcohol into the atmosphere, tubes should be filled completely and not uncapped prior to delivery to the laboratory. Blood alcohol levels are frequently collected in gray stopper tubes; however, laboratory protocol should be strictly followed.

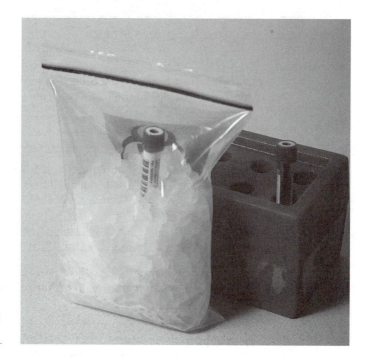

FIGURE 5–4. Specimens placed in a crushed ice and water slurry and an ice block.

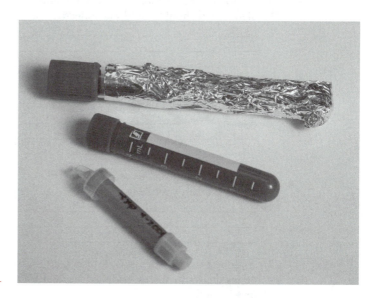

FIGURE 5–5. Specimens protected from light.

Special Venipuncture Collection Exercise

1. An outpatient comes to the collection station at 1300 with a requisition for a cardiac risk profile. What should the blood collector ask the patient before collecting the specimen?

   _____
   _____
   _____

2. Requisitions are received requesting that specimens for hemoglobin and hematocrit be collected at 0800, 1200, 1600, and 2000 from a patient on a medical-surgical unit. Is there a reason for these requests and, if so, what is it?

   _____
   _____
   _____

3. An outpatient comes to the collection area with a requisition for a fasting blood sugar (FBS) and 2-hour pp glucose. What procedure should be followed?

   _____
   _____
   _____

4. A patient receiving a 3-hour GTT vomits 20 minutes before the 3-hour specimen is scheduled. What should the blood collector do?

   _____
   _____
   _____

5. A cortisol level is ordered on a patient scheduled to go to physical therapy at 0900. How would this patient be scheduled? Explain your answer.

   _____
   _____
   _____

6. Would it be unusual to receive requests to collect theophylline levels at 0800 and again at 1200? Explain your answer.

   _____
   _____
   _____

7. A request to draw two sets of blood cultures within 30 minutes from a patient in the emergency department was made by the health-care provider. Is this a reasonable request? Why or why not?

   _____
   _____
   _____

8. One blood culture set was collected in a yellow stopper tubes and one in a lavender stopper tube and each transferred to bottles containing culture media. A known skin contaminant is cultured from one set.

   a. What errors in technique does this scenario indicate?

   _____

   _____

   _____

   b. Why was one culture negative?

   _____

   _____

   _____

9. Specimens for a stat ammonia level, a cold agglutinin test, and a complete blood count (CBC) were collected, each from a different patient in a different area of the unit. The three specimens were then sent to the laboratory in the pneumatic tube system. How will the quality of these test results be affected and why?

   _____

   _____

   _____

10. As the attorney for a defendant charged with having a blood alcohol level above the legal limit, you are questioning the health-care professional who collected the specimen.

   a. State three questions you would ask the blood collector to try to discredit the test result.

   _____

   _____

   _____

   b. How should a competent health-care professional answer these questions?

   _____

   _____

   _____

REVIEW QUESTIONS

1. The timing for a glucose tolerance test begins when:
   a. The fasting specimen is drawn
   b. The test results are completed on the fasting specimen
   c. The patient finishes drinking the glucose
   d. 30 minutes after the patient finishes drinking the glucose

2. Specimens are scheduled for collection at specific times for all of the following reasons EXCEPT:
   a. Measuring the body's metabolism of the test substance
   b. The substance exhibits diurnal variation
   c. Patients must be tested 2 hours before meals
   d. To determine blood levels of medications prior to the next dose

3. The trough level for therapeutic drug monitoring is collected:
   a. 30 minutes after the medication is administered
   b. 30 minutes before the medication is administered
   c. At the time specified by the manufacturer
   d. After the patient has fasted for 8 hours

4. The order in which cleansing solutions are applied to the patient's arm before and after the collection of a blood culture is:
   a. Soap, alcohol, and iodine
   b. Alcohol, iodine, and alcohol
   c. Iodine, alcohol, and soap
   d. Alcohol, alcohol, and iodine

5. True or False. Blood culture bottles and tubes contain an anticoagulant and must be mixed.

6. Two blood culture sets from a patient requiring ASAP administration of antibiotics are collected:
   a. Every 30 minutes
   b. Before, during, and after the antibiotic is administered
   c. Immediately from two different sites
   d. Before, during, and after the fever spikes

7. When blood is inoculated into blood culture bottles using a butterfly apparatus the:
   a. Anaerobic bottle is inoculated first
   b. Safety device is activated first
   c. Aerobic bottle is inoculated first
   d. Volume of blood inoculated is increased

8. Specimens that require chilling immediately after collection are placed in a:
   a. Container of ice cubes
   b. A container of crushed ice and water
   c. A bag of dry ice
   d. Flask of cold water

9. Specimens for cold agglutinins must be:
   a. Transported on ice
   b. Drawn in a green stopper tube
   c. Processed in a refrigerated centrifuge
   d. Kept warm

10. A falsely decreased blood alcohol level may be obtained if:
    a. Blood is collected in a gray stopper tube
    b. The site is cleansed with Zephiran Chloride
    c. The tube is only partially filled
    d. The tube is overfilled

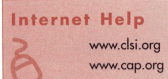

Internet Help

www.clsi.org

www.cap.org

Dermal Puncture

6

LEARNING OBJECTIVES

Upon completion of this unit, the reader will be able to:

- State the reasons for performing a dermal puncture.
- Describe the composition of capillary blood.
- Discuss the types of skin puncture devices available.
- Describe the types of microspecimen containers.
- Discuss the purpose and methodology for puncture site warming.
- Identify the acceptable site for performing heel and finger punctures.
- List four unacceptable areas for performing heel puncture.
- State the complications produced by the presence of alcohol at the puncture site.
- State the correct positioning of the lancet for dermal puncture.
- Explain why controlling the depth of the incision is important.
- Name the major cause of microspecimen contamination.
- State the order of collection for dermal puncture specimens.
- Describe the correct labeling of micro-specimens.

Introduction

Advances in laboratory instrumentation and the popularity of point-of-care testing have made it possible to perform a majority of laboratory tests on microsamples of blood obtained by dermal puncture on both pediatric and adult patients. This unit presents the required equipment and correct procedure necessary for dermal punctures to provide quality specimens.

Dermal puncture is the method of choice for collecting blood from infants and children younger than 2 years of age. Locating superficial veins large enough to accept even a small-gauge needle is difficult in these patients, and veins that are available may need to be reserved for IV therapy. Use of deep veins, such as the femoral vein, can be dangerous and may cause complications including cardiac arrest, venous thrombosis, hemorrhage, damage to surrounding tissue and organs, infection, reflex arteriospasm (which can possibly result in gangrene), and injury caused by restraining the child. Drawing excessive amounts of blood from premature and small infants can rapidly cause anemia, because a 2-lb infant may have a total blood volume of only 150 mL.

93

In adults, dermal puncture may be required for a variety of reasons, including:

1. Burned or scarred patients
2. Patients receiving chemotherapy who require frequent tests and whose veins must be reserved for therapy
3. Patients with thrombotic tendencies
4. Geriatric or other patients with very fragile veins
5. Patients with inaccessible veins
6. Home glucose monitoring and point-of-care testing

It may not be possible to obtain a satisfactory specimen by dermal puncture from patients who are severely dehydrated or who have poor peripheral circulation or who have swollen fingers. The interstitial fluid in a swollen finger may dilute the blood specimen if a finger stick is performed. Certain tests may not be collected by dermal puncture because of the larger amount of blood required; these include some coagulation studies, erythrocyte sedimentation rates, and blood cultures.

Importance of Correct Collection

Correct collection techniques are critical because of the smaller amount of blood that is collected and the higher possibility of specimen contamination, microclots, and hemolysis. Hemolysis is more frequently seen in specimens collected by dermal puncture than it is in those collected by venipuncture. Excessive squeezing of the puncture site to obtain enough blood is often the cause of hemolysis. The presence of hemolysis may not be detected in specimens containing bilirubin, but it interferes not only with the tests routinely affected by hemolysis, but also with the frequently requested neonatal bilirubin determination.

TECHNICAL TIP

Turn off the bili light when collecting specimens for neonatal bilirubin tests.

TECHNICAL TIP

By documenting that the specimen was collected by dermal puncture, the health-care provider can consider the collection technique when interpreting results.

Composition of Capillary Blood

Blood collected by dermal puncture comes from the capillaries, arterioles, and venules and may also contain small amounts of tissue (interstitial) fluid. Because of arterial pressure, the composition of this blood more closely resembles arterial blood than venous blood. With the exception of arterial blood gases (ABGs), few chemical differences exist between arterial and venous blood. The concentration of glucose is higher in blood obtained by dermal puncture than it is in blood obtained by venipuncture, and the concentrations of potassium, total protein, and calcium are lower. Alternating between dermal puncture and venipuncture should not be done when results are to be compared. Note on the requisition form if the specimen is from a dermal puncture.

Dermal Puncture Equipment

Dermal puncture supplies include automatic retractable safety puncture devices, microsample collection containers, 70-percent isopropyl alcohol pads, gauze pads, bandages, an approved sharps container, heel warmers, marking pen, glass slides, and gloves. With the exception of puncture devices, collection containers, heel warmers, and glass slides, the same equipment also is used for venipuncture (**Fig. 6–1**).

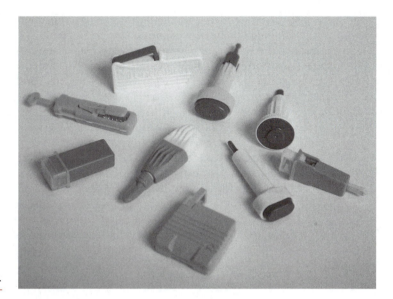

FIGURE 6–1. Dermal puncture devices.

Skin Puncture Devices

A variety of skin puncture devices are available in varying lengths and depths (**see Fig. 6–1**). All devices must have Occupational Safety & Health Administration (OSHA) required safety devices, such as retractable blades that are recommended to avoid possible exposure to blood-borne pathogens. To prevent contact with bone, the depth of the puncture produced by a device is critical. The incision depth of a skin puncture should be 2.0 to 2.5 mm for adults and should not exceed 2.0 mm for infants and small children. Manufacturers provide separate devices designed for heel sticks on premature infants, newborns, and babies and finger sticks on children and adults. The length of the lancets and the spring release mechanisms control the puncture depth with automatic devices. Punctures should never be performed using a surgical blade.

To produce adequate blood flow, the depth of the puncture is actually less important than the width of the puncture. As shown in **Figure 6–2,** the major vascular area of the skin is located at the dermal-subcutaneous juncture. The depth of this juncture can range from 0.35 to 1.6 mm in newborns to 3.0 mm in a large adult. Designated puncture devices easily reach it. Therefore, the number of severed capillaries depends on the width of the incision. Sufficient blood flow should be obtained from incision widths no larger than 2.5 mm.

FIGURE 6–2. Vascular area of the skin. *(Adapted from product literature, Becton, Dickinson, Franklin Lakes, NJ.)*

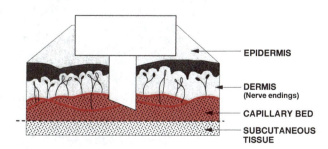

EPIDERMIS

DERMIS
(Nerve endings)

CAPILLARY BED

SUBCUTANEOUS
TISSUE

Color-coded lancets indicating the varying depths and widths to accommodate low, medium, and high blood flow requirements are available. The type of device selected depends on the age of the patient, the amount of blood specimen required, the collection site, and the puncture depth. BD Microtainer Genie Lancets (Becton Dickinson, Franklin Lakes, NJ) are available in a full range of blades for microhematocrit tubes and Microtainer blood collection tubes and needles to collect blood for single-drop glucose testing (**Fig. 6–3**). The BD Microtainer Contact-Activated Lancet is designed to activate only when the blade or needle is positioned and pressed against the skin. The BD Quikheel Lancets are color-coded heel-stick lancets made specifically for premature infants, newborns, and babies (**Fig. 6–4**).

International Technidyne Corporation (Edison, NJ) provides a range of color-coded fully automated, single-use, retractable, disposable devices in varying depths. Tenderfoot and Tenderlett devices are designed for heel and finger punctures, respectively. Models are available ranging from the Tenderfoot for preemies to the Tenderlett for adults.

Laser lancets (Lasette Plus, Cell Robotics International, Inc., Albuquerque, NM) are available for clinical and home use, and are approved by the Food and Drug Administration (FDA)

**Orange Genie™
Needle Lancet**
Designed for
glucose testing

**Pink Genie™
Lancet**
Designed to fill a
hematocrit tube and to
yield a drop of blood
for glucose testing

**Green Genie™
Lancet**
Designed to fill a BD™
microcollection tube

**Blue Genie™
Lancet**
Designed to fill a BD™
microcollection tube

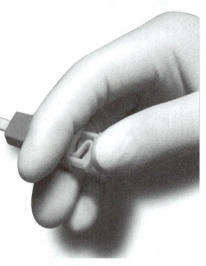

FIGURE 6–3. Genie safety lancet. *(Courtesy of Becton Dickinson, Franklin Lakes, NJ.)*

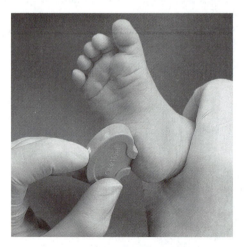

FIGURE 6–4. Quikheel lancet. *(Courtesy of Becton Dickinson, Franklin Lakes, NJ.)*

for adults and children older than 5 years of age. The lightweight, portable, battery-operated device eliminates the risks of accidental punctures and the need for sharps containers. A single-use disposable insert prevents cross-contamination between patients. The laser light penetrates the skin 1 to 2 mm, producing a small hole in the capillary bed by vaporizing water in the skin. This creates a smaller wound, reduces the pain and soreness associated with capillary puncture, and allows up to 100 μL of blood to be collected (**Fig. 6–5**).

Microspecimen Containers

Figure 6–6 illustrates some of the major specimen containers available for collection of microsamples, including capillary tubes, micropipettes, microcollection tubes, and micropipettes with dilution systems. Some containers are designated for a specific test, and others serve multiple purposes.

FIGURE 6–5. Laser lancet, the Lasette Plus. *(From Strasinger, SK, and Di Lorenzo, MS: Phlebotomy Workbook, ed. 2. FA Davis, Philadelphia, 2003, Figure 9–6, p. 189, with permission. Courtesy of Cell Robotics, Inc., Albuquerque, NM.)*

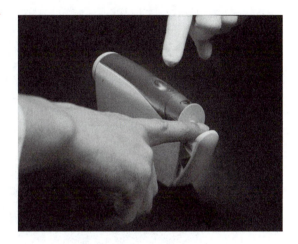

FIGURE 6–6. Microspecimen containers.

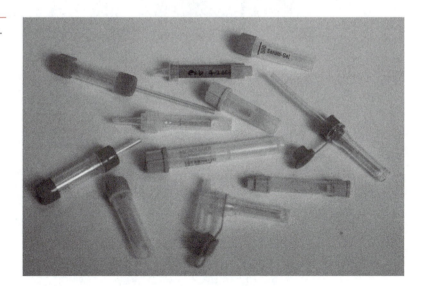

CAPILLARY TUBES

Capillary tubes, frequently referred to as microhematocrit tubes, are small plastic tubes that fill by capillary action and are used to collect approximately 50 to 75 μL of blood for the primary purpose of performing a microhematocrit. The tubes are designed to fit into a hematocrit centrifuge and its corresponding hematocrit reader. Tubes are available plain or coated with ammonium heparin and are color-coded with a red band for heparinized tubes and a blue band for plain tubes. Heparinized tubes should be used for hematocrits collected by dermal puncture, and plain tubes are used when the test is being performed on previously anticoagulated blood. When sufficient blood has been collected, the end of the capillary tube that has not been used to collect the specimen is closed with a clay sealant or a plastic plug. Tubes protected by plastic sleeves and self-sealing tubes are available to prevent breakage when collecting specimens and sealing the microcapillary tubes (**Fig. 6–7**).

MICROPIPETTES

Larger capillary tubes, called Caraway or Natelson pipets, are used when tests other than a microhematocrit are requested. The pipets have a tapered end for specimen collection and fill by capillary action. Pipet lengths vary from 75 mm for Caraway pipets to 220 to 420 mm for Natelson pipets. Pipets are available plain or with ammonium heparin and are color-coded, respectively, with blue or red bands. After collection of the sample, the nontapered ends are sealed with specifically matched soft plastic caps or clay sealant. Tubes designed for capillary blood gas specimens are also available.

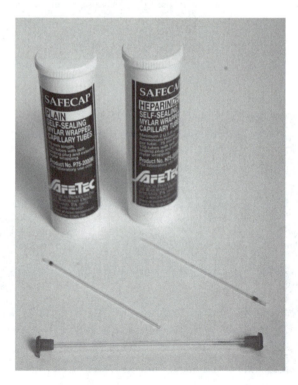

FIGURE 6–7. Capillary tubes and a micropipette.

MICROCOLLECTION TUBES

Plastic collection tubes such as the BD Microtainer Tube (Becton, Dickinson, Franklin Lakes, NJ) provide a larger collection volume. A variety of anticoagulants and additives, including separator gel, are available, and the tubes are color-coded in the same way as evacuated tubes. Amber-colored PST and SST Microtainers are available for light-sensitive analyte testing. Some tubes are supplied with a capillary scoop collector top that is replaced by a color-coded plastic sealer top after the specimen is collected. Microtainer tubes are designed to hold approximately 600 µL of blood. BD Microtainer tubes with BD Microguard closures are designed to reduce the risk of blood splatter and blood leakage. The Microguard closure is removed by twisting and lifting. Tubes have a wide diameter, textured interior, and an integrated blood collection scoop to enhance blood flow into the tube and eliminate the need to assemble the equipment. After completion of the collection of blood, the cap is placed on the container, and anticoagulated tubes are gently inverted 10 to 20 times to ensure complete mixing. Tubes have markings to indicate minimum and maximum collection amounts to prevent underfilling or overfilling that could cause erroneous results. Tube extenders are available for this system to facilitate labeling and handling (**see Fig. 6–6**). Separation of serum or plasma is achieved by centrifugation in specifically designed centrifuges.

Other capillary blood collection devices have plastic capillary tubes inserted into the collection container (SAFE-T-FILL capillary blood collection system, RAM Scientific Co., Needham, MA). After blood has been collected, the capillary tube is removed and the appropriate color-coded cap closes the tube.

MICROPIPET AND DILUTION SYSTEM

The Unopette system (Becton, Dickinson, Franklin Lakes, NJ) is designed for tests that can be performed on diluted whole blood, primarily white blood cell and platelet tests. The system consists of a sealed plastic reservoir containing a measured amount of diluent, a calibrated capillary pipette, and a plastic pipet shield. The amount and type of diluent and the size of the capillary pipette correspond to the specific test to be run. Pipets are designed to collect only the amount of blood for which they are calibrated (**Fig. 6–8**).

Dermal Puncture Procedure

Many of the procedures associated with venipuncture also apply to dermal puncture; therefore, major emphasis in this unit is on the techniques and complications that are unique to dermal puncture.

Prepuncture Preparation

TECHNICAL TIP

Consider giving parents the option to stay with a child or leave the room.

The requisition provides the information as to the age of the patient and the test requested. This determines which of the variety of puncture devices and collection containers should be used for the dermal puncture. Patient identification may require confirmation from a parent or guardian. When a specimen is collected by dermal puncture, it must be noted on the requisition form, because the concentration of some substances differs in venous and capillary blood.

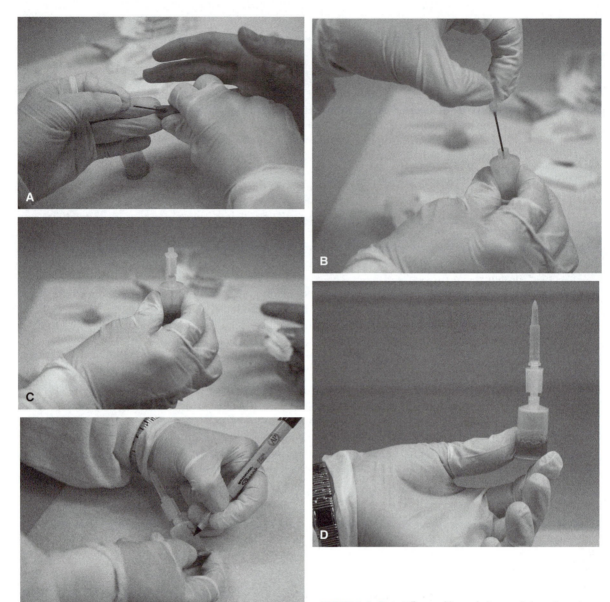

FIGURE 6–8 *A.* Filling calibrated pipette. *B.* Inserting pipette into diluting fluid. *C.* Rinsing the pipette and mixing blood with diluting fluid. *D.* Mixed Unopette. *E.* Labeling Unopette.

Patient Preparation

For optimum blood flow, the area to be punctured should be warm. This is primarily a concern for patients with very cold or cyanotic fingers, for heel sticks to collect multiple samples, and for the collection of capillary blood gases. Warming dilates the blood vessels and increases arterial blood flow. Warming is performed by moistening a towel with warm water (42°C) or by activating a commercial heel warmer and covering the site for 3 to 5 minutes.

Site Selection

The choice of a puncture area is based on the age and size of the patient. Select puncture sites that provide sufficient distance between the skin and the bone to avoid accidental contact with the bone that may cause infection (osteomyelitis). The primary sites are the heel and the distal segments of the third and fourth fingers. Performing dermal punctures on earlobes is usually not recommended.

Areas selected for dermal puncture should not be callused, scarred, bruised, edematous, cold or cyanotic, or infected. Punctures should never be made through previous puncture sites, because this can easily introduce microorganisms into the puncture and allow them to reach the bone. Do not collect blood from the fingers on the side of a mastectomy without a physician's order.

HEEL PUNCTURE SITES

The heel is the most common site for dermal punctures on infants younger than 1 year of age, because it contains more tissue than the fingers and has not yet become callused from walking. Acceptable areas for heel puncture are shown in **Figure 6–9** and are described as the medial and lateral areas of the bottom (plantar) surface of the heel. These areas can be determined by drawing imaginary lines extending back from the middle of the large toe and from between the fourth and fifth toes. It is in these areas that the distance between the skin and the heel bone (calcaneus) is greatest. Notice the short distance between the back (posterior curvature) of the heel and the calcaneus. This is the reason that this area is never acceptable for heel puncture.

Punctures should not be performed in other areas of the foot, and particularly not in the arch, where they may cause damage to nerves and tendons.

FINGER PUNCTURE SITES

Finger punctures are performed on adults and children older than 1 year of age. Fingers of infants younger than 1 year old may not contain enough tissue to prevent contact with the bone.

The fleshy areas located near the center of the third and fourth fingers on the palmar side are the sites of choice for finger puncture (**Fig. 6–10**). Because the tip and sides of the finger contain only about half the tissue mass of the central area, the possibility of bone injury is increased in these areas. Problems associated with the use of other fingers include possible calluses on the thumb, increased nerve endings in the index finger, and decreased tissue in the fifth finger.

SUMMARY OF DERMAL PUNCTURE SITE SELECTION

1. Use the medial and lateral areas of the plantar surface of the heel.
2. Use the central fleshy area of the third or fourth fingers.
3. Do not use the fingers on the side of a mastectomy.
4. Do not use the back of the heel.
5. Do not use the arch of the foot.
6. Do not puncture through old sites.
7. Do not use areas with visible damage.

HEEL PUNCTURE SITES

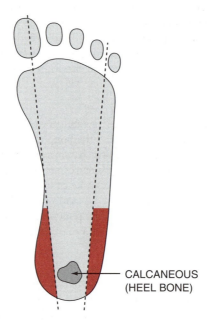

CALCANEOUS
(HEEL BONE)

FIGURE 6–9. Acceptable heel puncture sites. *(From Strasinger, SK, and Di Lorenzo, MS: Phlebotomy Workbook, ed. 2. FA Davis, Philadelphia, 2003, Figure 9–9, p. 192, with permission.)*

■ PUNCTURE ZONE

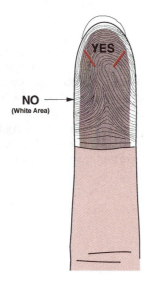

NO
(White Area)

YES

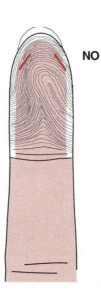

NO

FIGURE 6–10. Acceptable finger puncture sites and correct puncture angle. *(From Strasinger, SK, and Di Lorenzo, MS: Phlebotomy Workbook, ed. 2. FA Davis, Philadelphia, 2003, Figure 9–10, p. 192, with permission.)*

TECHNICAL TIP

Use of povidone-iodine is not recommended for dermal punctures because specimen contamination may elevate some test results, including bilirubin, phosphorus, uric acid, and potassium.

Cleansing the Site

The selected site is cleansed with 70-percent isopropyl alcohol using a circular motion (**Fig. 6–12A**). The alcohol should be allowed to dry on the skin for maximum bacteriostatic action, and the residue removed with gauze to prevent possible interference with test results. Failure to allow the alcohol to dry will:

1. Cause a stinging sensation for the patient.
2. Contaminate the specimen.
3. Hemolyze red blood cells (RBCs).
4. Prevent formation of a rounded blood drop because blood will mix with the alcohol and run down the finger.

Performing the Puncture

While the puncture is performed, the heel or finger should be well supported and held firmly, without squeezing the puncture area. Massaging the area before the puncture may increase blood flow to the area. The heel is held between the thumb and index finger of the nondominant hand (**Fig. 6–11**). The finger is held between the thumb and index finger with the palmar surface facing up and the finger pointing downward to increase blood flow.

TECHNICAL TIP

Failure to place puncture devices firmly on the skin is the primary cause of insufficient blood flow. One firm puncture is less painful for the patient than two "mini" punctures.

Place the puncture device firmly on the puncture site. Do not indent the skin when placing the lancet on the puncture site. The blade of the lancet should be aligned to cut across (perpendicular to) the grooves of the finger or heel print (**Fig. 6–12B**). This prevents the blood from running into the grooves that prevent the formation of a rounded drop of blood (**see Fig. 6–10**). Depress the lancet and hold for a moment, then release. Pressure must be maintained, because the elasticity of the skin naturally inhibits penetration of the blade. Removal of the lancet before the puncture is complete will yield a low blood flow.

After completing the puncture, the lancet should be placed in an approved sharps container. A new puncture device must be used if an additional puncture is required.

FIGURE 6–11. Correct position for heel puncture. *(From Strasinger, SK, and Di Lorenzo, MA: Phlebotomy Workbook, ed. 2. FA Davis, Philadelphia, 2003, Figure 9–11, p. 193, with permission.)*

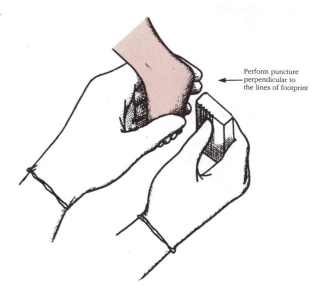

Perform puncture perpendicular to the lines of footprint

Specimen Collection

Before beginning the collection, wipe away the first drop of blood with sterile gauze (**Fig. 6–12C**). This will prevent contamination of the specimen with residual alcohol and tissue fluid released during the puncture. Some point-of-care instruments do not require that the first drop of blood be wiped away. Always follow the manufacturer's instructions. When collecting microspecimens, even a minute amount of contamination can severely affect the sample quality. Therefore, blood should be flowing freely from the puncture site as a result of firm pressure and should not be obtained by milking or strenuous massaging of the surrounding tissue that will release tissue fluid. The most satisfactory blood flow is obtained by alternately applying and releasing pressure to the area. Tightly squeezing the area with no relaxation will cut off blood flow to the puncture site.

Because collection containers fill by capillary action, the collection tip can be lightly touched to the drop of blood and the blood will be drawn into the container. Collection devices should not touch the puncture site and should not be scraped over the skin, because this will produce specimen contamination and hemolysis. Fingers are positioned slightly downward with the palmar surface also facing slightly down during the collection procedure. To prevent introduction of air bubbles, capillary tubes and micropipets are held horizontally while being filled. The presence of air bubbles limits the amount of blood that can be collected per tube and interferes with blood gas determinations and tests performed with Unopettes. When the tubes are filled, they are sealed with sealant clay or designated plastic caps.

Microcollection tubes are slanted down during the collection, and blood is allowed to run through the capillary collection scoop and down the side of the tube. The tip of the collection container is placed beneath the puncture site and touches the underside of the drop (**Fig. 6–12D**). The first 3 drops of blood provide the channel to allow blood to flow freely into the container. Gently tapping the bottom of the tube may be necessary to force blood to the bottom. When a tube is filled, the color-coded top is attached (**Fig. 6–12E**). Tubes with anticoagulants should be inverted 10 to 20 times. If blood flow is slow, it may be necessary to mix the tube while the collection is in progress. It is important to work quickly, because blood that takes more than 2 minutes to collect may form microclots in an anticoagulated Microtainer.

ORDER OF COLLECTION

The order of draw for collecting multiple specimens from a dermal puncture is important because of the tendency of platelets to accumulate at the site of a wound. Blood to be used for tests for the evaluation of platelets, such as blood smear, platelet count, and complete blood count (CBC), must be collected first. The blood smear should be made first, followed by specimens for the Unopette system or the lavender EDTA Microtainer, other anticoagulated Microtainers, and then serum Microtainers.

TECHNICAL TIP

Applying pressure about ½ inch away from the puncture site frequently produces better blood flow than pressure very close to the site.

TECHNICAL TIP

While collecting the sample, the patient's hand does not have to be completely turned over. Rotating the hand 90 degrees allows blood collectors to clearly see the blood drops without placing themselves in awkward positions.

TECHNICAL TIP

Strong consistant squeezing (milking) must be avoided as it can cause hemolysis or tissue-fluid contamination of the specimen.

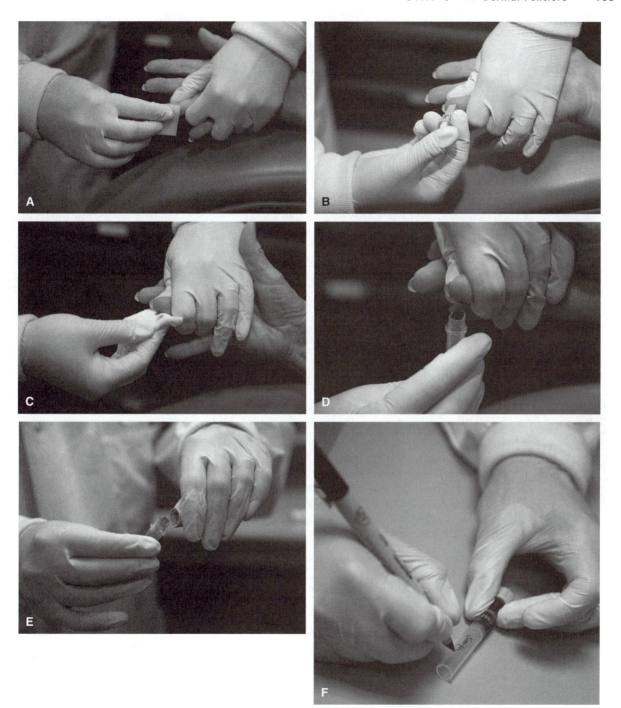

FIGURE 6–12 *A.* Cleansing the site. *B.* Puncturing the finger with an automatic safety lancet. *C.* Wiping away the first drop of blood. *D.* Collecting blood in a Microtainer. *E.* Capping the Microtainer for inversion. *F.* Labeling the Microtainer (note extender).

Bandaging the Patient

When sufficient blood has been collected, pressure is applied to the puncture site with gauze. The finger or heel is elevated and pressure is applied until the bleeding stops. Confirm that the bleeding has stopped before removing the pressure.

Bandages are not used for children younger than 2 years of age because they may remove the bandages, place them in their mouths, and possibly aspirate the bandages. The adhesive may also cause irritation to sensitive skin, particularly the fragile skin of a newborn or older adult patient.

Labeling the Specimen

Microsamples must be labeled with the same information required for venipuncture specimens. Labels can be wrapped around microcollection tubes or groups of capillary pipets. For transport, capillary pipettes are then placed in a large tube, because the outside of the capillary pipets may be contaminated with blood.

Becton Dickinson Microtainer collection tubes have extenders that can be attached to the container. This allows the computer label to be applied vertically (**Fig. 6-12F**).

Completion of the Procedure

The dermal puncture procedure is completed by disposing of all used materials in appropriate containers, removing gloves, washing hands, and thanking the patient and/or the parents for their cooperation.

All special handling procedures associated with venipuncture specimens also apply to microspecimens.

To prevent excessive removal of blood from small infants, a log sheet for documenting the amount of blood collected each time a procedure is requested may be required by institutional policy.

As with venipuncture, it is recommended that only two punctures be attempted to collect the blood. When a second puncture must be made to collect the sufficient amount of blood, the blood should not be added to the previously collected tube. This can cause erroneous results due to microclots and hemolysis.

TECHNICAL TIP

Clotting is triggered immediately on skin puncture and represents the greatest obstacle in collecting quality specimens.

Summary of the Dermal Puncture Procedure

1. Obtain and examine the requisition form.
2. Assemble equipment and supplies.
3. Greet the patient and/or the parents.
4. Identify the patient.
5. Position the patient and the parents.
6. Wash hands and put on gloves.
7. Select the puncture site.
8. Warm the puncture site if necessary.
9. Cleanse and allow the puncture site to dry.
10. Prepare equipment.
11. Perform the puncture.
12. Dispose of the puncture device.
13. Wipe away the first drop of blood.
14. Make blood smears if requested.

15. Collect the hematology specimen and then other specimens.
16. Mix the specimens if necessary.
17. Apply pressure.
18. Label the specimens.
19. Perform appropriate specimen handling.
20. Examine the site for stoppage of bleeding.
21. Apply bandage if the patient is over 2 years of age.
22. Thank the patient and/or the parents.
23. Dispose of used supplies.
24. Remove and dispose of gloves.
25. Wash hands.
26. Complete any required paperwork.
27. Deliver specimens to the appropriate locations.

Dermal Puncture Collection Exercise

1. The phlebotomy supervisor is informed that many of the specimens collected by the personnel in the pediatric outpatient unit are hemolyzed. The supervisor schedules a continuing education in-service for the unit.

   a. Why should preparation of the collection site be stressed?

   _____
   _____
   _____

   b. Why is it important for the personnel to obtain rounded drops of blood to prevent hemolysis?

   _____
   _____
   _____

   c. Should the in-service include the procedure to follow when a second puncture must be performed to obtain a full tube of blood? Why or why not?

   _____
   _____
   _____

2. During a dermal puncture in-service, the instructor noticed that a blood collector was having difficulty obtaining rounded drops of blood. Why should the instructor check the following parts of the blood collector's technique?

   a. Site cleansing

   _____
   _____
   _____

   b. Alignment of the puncture device

   _____
   _____
   _____

c. Puncture technique

_____
_____
_____

d. Application of pressure

_____
_____
_____

3. The blood collector delivers a lavender top Microtainer and a red top Microtainer to the laboratory. The hematology supervisor is concerned because the platelet count was decreased but the other CBC parameters were within the normal range. Platelet clumping was noticed on the peripheral blood smear.

a. Could the blood collection technique have caused this?

_____

b. Why or why not?

_____
_____

Evaluation of a Finger Stick

Rating System   2 = Satisfactory   1 = Needs Improvement   0 = Incorrect/Did Not Perform

_____ **1.** Greets patient and explains procedure.	_____ **14.** Disposes of puncture device in sharps container.
_____ **2.** Examines requisition form.	
_____ **3.** Asks patient to state full name.	_____ **15.** Wipes away first drop of blood.
_____ **4.** Compares requisition information and patient's statement.	_____ **16.** Collects two microhematocrit tubes without air bubbles.
_____ **5.** Compares requisition information with ID band.	_____ **17.** Seals tubes.
	_____ **18.** Applies gauze to site and asks patient to apply pressure.
_____ **6.** Washes hands and puts on gloves.	_____ **19.** Labels tubes and confirms the information with the ID band or patient.
_____ **7.** Organizes and assembles equipment.	
_____ **8.** Selects appropriate finger.	_____ **20.** Examines site for stoppage of bleeding and applies bandage.
_____ **9.** Warms finger if necessary.	
_____ **10.** Gently massages finger.	_____ **21.** Thanks patient.
_____ **11.** Cleanses site with alcohol and allows it to air dry.	_____ **22.** Disposes of used supplies.
_____ **12.** Does not contaminate puncture device.	_____ **23.** Removes gloves.
_____ **13.** Smoothly performs puncture across fingerprint.	_____ **24.** Washes hands.

Total points
Maximum points = 48
COMMENTS

REVIEW QUESTIONS

1. When selecting a dermal puncture device, the most critical consideration is the:
   a. Width of the incision
   b. Amount of blood needed
   c. Depth of the incision
   d. Tests requested

2. Dermal puncture specimens are collected in all of the following EXCEPT:
   a. Pediatric evacuated tubes
   b. Microhematocrit tubes
   c. Microtainer tubes
   d. Unopettes

3. All of the following are acceptable skin puncture devices EXCEPT:
   a. Genie lancets
   b. Surgical blades
   c. Laser lancets
   d. Tenderfoots

4. Capillary punctures on newborns are performed on the:
   a. Index finger
   b. Plantar area of the heel
   c. Back of the heel
   d. Earlobe

5. Failure to allow the alcohol to dry on the puncture site may cause:
   a. Inability to form a rounded drop
   b. Specimen contamination
   c. Red blood cell hemolysis
   d. All of the above

6. Wiping away the first drop of blood:
   a. Increases blood flow
   b. Prevents specimen contamination
   c. Causes air bubbles to enter the tube
   d. Stimulates platelets and faster clotting

7. The possibility of infection is increased when:
   a. The thumb is punctured
   b. Alcohol is used to cleanse the site
   c. A puncture is made through a previous site
   d. The palmar side of the finger is punctured

8. Failure to puncture across the fingerprint during a finger puncture will cause:
   a. Blood to run down the finger
   b. Hemolysis
   c. Contamination of the specimen
   d. Additional patient discomfort

9. Selection of an improper heel puncture site can result in:
   a. Puncture of the calcaneous
   b. Specimen hemolysis
   c. The need for vigorous massaging
   d. Increased blood flow

10. The order of draw for a bilirubin, blood smear, and CBC by dermal puncture is:
    a. CBC, blood smear, and bilirubin
    b. Blood smear, CBC, and bilirubin
    c. Bilirubin, blood smear, and CBC
    d. Blood smear, bilirubin, and CBC

Internet Help

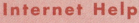

www.bd.com   www.itcmed.com
www.clsi.org   www.cellrobotics.com

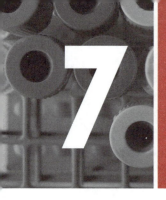

7 Point-of-Care Testing

Introduction

Point-of-care testing (POCT) is laboratory testing performed at or near the patient bedside. POCT also may be referred to as "near patient testing," "bedside testing," POCT, or POC. Although POCT is laboratory testing, the majority of POCT is performed by nonlaboratory personnel. POCT personnel, also referred to as "operators," are usually primary patient providers. This group of operators includes nurses, respiratory therapists, physicians, medical and nursing assistants, and other health-care professionals. POCT is used in many patient care settings including emergency departments, intensive care units, surgical suites, radiology, physician office clinics, health fairs, dialysis units, and other health-care settings.

As technology has advanced, the scope of POCT and its role in providing quality patient care has expanded at an exponential rate. **Table 7–1** lists commonly performed POCTs and their associated laboratory section.

Manufacturers have continued to expand the list of available POCTs and the sample types that can be analyzed. Whole blood, plasma, urine samples, and direct swabs from an infected area are still the most common sample types, but saliva and other body fluids also are being used. Some newer technologies do not require a specimen, such as the devices that perform transcutaneous bilirubin and noninvasive glucose testing. These technologies are capable of obtaining a laboratory answer by placing the POCT device directly on the patient's skin without obtaining a sample from the patient. The rapid growth of POCT technology has provided health-care professionals the mobility to bring a large test menu of rapid laboratory services to the patient's bedside. Other advantages to POCT may include decreased turn-around-time (TAT) for test results, decreased specimen volume, reduction or elimination of specimen transport to the main laboratory, simple testing procedure (ease of use), decreased

TABLE 7–1. Common POCTs Associated With Laboratory Departments

LABORATORY DEPARTMENT	TESTS
Hematology	Hemoglobin
	Hematocrit
	Erythrocyte sedimentation rate (ESR)
Chemistry	Glucose, arterial blood gases (ABGs), lipid panels, blood urea nitrogen (BUN), electrolytes, comprehensive metabolic profile, cardiac markers, liver function, human chorionic gonadotropin, hemoglobin A1c
Serology	Human immunodeficiency virus,
	Mononucleosis, *Helicobacter pylori*
Urinalysis and Body Fluids	Reagent strip urinalysis, occult blood, Gastroccult, body fluid pH
Urine Toxicology (drugs of abuse)	Amphetamines, marijuana, cocaine, benzodiazepines, barbiturates, ethanol
Microbiology	Group A Streptococcus, influenza A/B, respiratory syncytial virus (RSV)
Coagulation	Prothrombin time (PT)/international normalizing ratio (INR), activated partial thromboplastin time (APTT), activated clotting time (ACT)

analyzer size, and increased opportunity for more personal patient interaction with nursing or other designated care providers.

POCT also has several identified drawbacks. Because POCT is true laboratory testing, it also is governed by all of the same regulations that apply to laboratory testing performed in a traditional laboratory. Accreditation requirements, charging and billing mechanisms, documentation of patient results, quality control (QC) testing and documentation, and inventory management are all processes that can be problematic. In many settings, a large number of patient care providers perform POCTs compared with a much smaller number of laboratory staff that would be performing the test in a traditional laboratory setting. The large number of operators can have a dilution effect on operator competency. This is particularly apparent when the volume of POCTs is low and the number of operators is high. The operators have fewer opportunities to maintain their skill level, since the test is performed at a very low frequency.

POCT technology benefits also have been realized in many traditional laboratory settings. Decreased specimen volume, small analyzer size and portability, ease of use, and fast TAT have made POCT technology a replacement option for laboratory equipment in many traditional laboratories.

TECHNICAL TIP

Tests are continually being developed. For an up-to-date listing of POCTs, refer to www.cms.hhs.gov/CLIA/.

Phases of Laboratory Testing

Laboratory testing is performed in three phases. These are referred to as preanalytic, analytic, and postanalytic. Procedures should be available to the testing operators that address all three phases of testing for each test. The preanalytic phase encompasses the test ordering process, patient identification and patient preparation, specimen collection and handling, reagent storage, and preparing materials, equipment, and the testing area. The analytic phase is when the actual test is performed, and also includes QC testing, and result interpretation. The final post-analytic phase involves recording and reporting results, addressing critical values when indicated, following through for confirmatory testing, and biohazard waste disposal. All three phases are vitally important to quality patient testing.

It is important to note that the majority of all laboratory testing errors occur in the preanalytic and postanalytic phases of testing. Because the technology for most POCT is designed to be user-friendly, the potential of performing a test incorrectly and the direct impact of that error is often underestimated. POCT traditionally provides a very short TAT from the collection of the sample to the time a result is obtained. Throughout the very brief testing process, care must be taken throughout all three phases of testing to ensure a timely, quality test result every time. Failure to address just one of several critical steps in each testing process can lead to a negative patient outcome brought about by reporting a fast, but incorrect, result.

> **TECHNICAL TIP**
>
> Patient identification must be verified at the bedside and entered correctly in the POCT device.

Preanalytic Phase

Patient identification is the primary concern prior to performing any laboratory test. Due to the nature of POCT, many times no collection tube or sample cup is required to contain the specimen prior to performing the test. Although this is perceived as an advantage and can decrease the time it takes to perform a test, it also eliminates one of the traditional audit trails used to verify positive patient identification. Many new POCT devices enable the operator to enter the patient identification into the POCT device, so that the information is captured and stored electronically. Newer technology also has the ability to capture patient identification and operator identification using a bar-code scanner. Failure to identify the patient correctly in the POCT device can result in failure to document a test result that was used to treat or not treat a patient, or the results may be reported on the wrong patient. Both of these scenarios could result in a negative outcome for the patient.

> **TECHNICAL TIP**
>
> Careful attention to collection technique and sample application to the test device is critical for POC coagulation testing.

Other preanalytic variables that can affect patient outcomes include correct specimen collection and proper storage of equipment and supplies. Many POCT supplies have very specific storage requirements. Many are sensitive to heat, light, and moisture. Others require refrigeration and warm-up to room temperature prior to use. The expiration date for some testing supplies changes when moved from refrigerated storage to room temperature, or whenever the primary container is opened. No testing supplies should be used past their expiration dates.

Analytic Phase

The analytic phase is the phase when the actual test is performed. For all POCT, it is imperative that manufacturers' instructions are followed. Application of the sample to the test device and test timing are common errors associated with the analytical phase. For some tests, especially coagulation methods, the time between the actual collection of the specimen and application to the POCT device is critical, since coagulation starts immediately after the blood sample is removed from the patient. Test methods that utilize a color formation are especially sensitive to critical timing. A test that is read too early or too late can be misinterpreted due to the lack of color development, color overdevelopment, or degradation of the color that is to be measured. Although POCT devices are designed to be portable, many cannot be moved when analyzing a specimen, since movement may disrupt the flow of specimen through the device.

Test interpretation is another part of the analytic phase. Many POCT devices, both automated and manual test kit methods, have built-in procedural QC mechanisms to monitor the analytic phase of testing and alert the operator that a test is invalid or the device simply does not display a test result. Kit methods often include a "control" line that aids in correct interpretation of the test. The presence of the control line indicates that the test was performed correctly. If the control line does not appear, the test is invalid and the patient result cannot be interpreted or reported. The invalid test may be caused by compromised integrity of the testing supplies or addition of test reagents in the wrong order.

POCT results can be qualitative, quantitative, or semiquantitative. Qualitative results are reported as positive or negative. A urine pregnancy test is an example of a qualitative test, since the result is reported as either positive or negative. Quantitative results are numeric results, such as a whole blood glucose result. Semiquantitative results are reported in terms of reaction intensity (1+, 2+, 3+) that equates to a range of numeric values.

Postanalytic Phase

The postanalytic phase of testing includes documentation of the results. Many POC devices have the capability to capture results electronically and transmit those results to the permanent medical record. Not all health-care facilities, however, are able to fully utilize these features.

Manual documentation of POCT results is not uncommon. When manual documentation is employed, duplicate transcription is often required to document the result in the patient's permanent medical record and on a laboratory log. The patient's name, unique identifier, date and time of result, testing operator, and test results are required documentation. Results are customarily reported with normal patient reference ranges, although it also is common to include therapeutic ranges for most coagulation results (**Fig. 7–1**). A written record of lot numbers and expiration dates for supplies also may be required, depending on the test complexity and accrediting organization (**Fig. 7–2**).

In some cases, even after the documentation is completed, the testing process is not finished. POCT staff also must be familiar with the critical values for each test and the processes for notification of attending staff and/or initiating treatment adjustments. For some POCTs, a result may require confirmatory testing. The confirmatory testing process may include obtaining an additional order, patient consent, and/or collection of a new specimen. Finally, the operator must properly dispose of all biohazard items.

TECHNICAL TIP

Incorrect patient results may be obtained if the critical test procedure is not followed.

TECHNICAL TIP

Follow manufacturers' storage requirements for reagent strips. Most testing strips may not be stored in an open container and exposed to light, moisture, or heat.

TECHNICAL TIP

When working for a different organization, do not assume that you will be using the same procedure kits. Read the package inserts for all kits and instruments before performing tests.

Quality Control

The purpose of QC is to ensure the accuracy, precision, and reliability of the test system. Specific QC information regarding the type of control specimen, preparation and handling, frequency of use, tolerance levels, and method of recording the QC results are included in the procedure for each test. QC procedures verify the functional integrity of the testing supplies and the POCT device. QC also confirms that the testing operator can perform the test correctly. Additionally, QC testing must be performed to satisfy regulatory requirements. Regulations governing all laboratory testing require that patient test results must correlate with QC results. This means that a laboratory must be able to prove that the reliability of the test system was confirmed each day a patient test was performed. Successful QC performance ensures that the operator can use the

LABORATORY REPORT FORM

Patient Name: _____   Test Date: _____

Patient ID: _____

Test	Results	Reference Ranges
Urinalysis (adult)	Clean Catch YES NO	
Specific gravity		1.001–1.030
pH		5–6
Leukocytes		Neg
Nitrate		Neg
Protein (mg/dL)	mg/dL	Neg
Glucose (mg/dL)	mg/dL	Neg
Ketone		Neg
Urobilinogen (mg/dL)	mg/dL	<1
Bilirubin		Neg
Blood (RBC/uL)	RBC/uL	Neg
Stool for Occult Blood	Internal Pos/Neg Controls: OK	Neg
Hemoglobin by HemoCue (g/dL)	g/dL	4 to 10 months 10.0–14.0 g/dL
		10 mo to 3 yrs 11.0–14.0 g/dL
		4 to 9 yrs 11.5–15.0 g/dL
		9 to 14 yrs 12.0–15.6 g/dL
		Adult Female 11.6–16.1 g/dL
		Adult Male 13.3–17.7 g/dL
Mono Test	Internal Pos/Neg Controls: OK	Neg
Rapid Strep A/Throat	Internal Pos/Neg Controls: OK	Neg
Glucose (Whole Blood)	mg/dL	70–99 mg/dL (fasting)
		If patient not fasting—
		Time of last food intake:
		Time of test: _____
Urine Pregnancy Test (hCG)	Internal Pos/Neg Controls: OK	Neg (LMP)
Vaginal Wet Prep/KOH		Neg
(PPMP, performed only by		
Nurse Practitioner)		
Comments:		

Person performing test (Initial): _____   Practitioner: _____

FIGURE 7–1. Laboratory report form with reference ranges.

SURESTEP WHOLE BLOOD GLUCOSE
PATIENT/QUALITY CONTROL LOG

Test Strip Lot # _____ Control Code: _____ Exp. Date: _____
Low Control Lot # _____ Low Control QC Range: _____ Exp. Date: _____
High Control Lot # _____ High Control QC Range: _____ Exp. Date: _____

DATE	PATIENT NAME (Or use patient label)	PATIENT ID	PATIENT RESULT	LOW CONTROL	HIGH CONTROL	TECH

Reviewed by: _____ **Date:** _____

FIGURE 7-2. SureStep whole blood glucose patient/QC log.

test system to perform patient testing and that the patient result will be valid. If the QC results are within the specified performance range, meaning the QC results are the expected answers, then the operator also can test a patient sample and get a quality result. The operator has controlled the quality of the test system.

There are two types of controls, external and internal. External QCs are tested in the same manner as a patient specimen. The external QC may challenge all three phases of testing, since it can address sample preparation, application, test performance, and result documentation. External QC solutions, also known as QC materials, are commonly used to verify test systems that use urine or blood sample types. Internal QCs are contained within the test system, and are sometimes referred to as procedural controls. Internal controls are commonly used in test kit systems, which verify that the test kit and any added reagents performed as expected. Some test systems also use another type of internal control called electronic QC (EQC). EQC uses a mechanical or electrical sample in place of a patient or liquid QC sample. This type of QC can be internal to the POCT device or an external component inserted into the POCT device. Although EQC can verify the functional ability of the POCT device, it does not verify the integrity of the testing supplies. Many test systems use a combination of external and internal controls to verify the entire test system is working properly. Many POCT devices have a safety feature that locks the meter to prevent any patient testing until the QC error (internal, external, and/or EQC) is resolved.

QC is often performed at scheduled times, such as daily or the beginning of each shift. At a minimum, two levels of QC materials, usually one normal and one abnormal sample, are required each day patient testing is performed. Two different levels of QC are used to assure the test system will measure normal and abnormal patient samples accurately. QC must be performed, and equally important, the results must be acceptable (within the expected range) before patient tests are performed or reported. External QC testing for POCT methods is often required each time a new test kit is opened, or with each new lot and each new shipment of testing supplies. Internal QC procedural controls are usually performed more frequently, and are often performed with each test. EQC is usually performed on a timed schedule, which can be daily, or every few hours, depending on the manufacturer's recommendations and laboratory regulations. Light, moisture, cleaning agents, or premature deterioration can affect POCT supplies. Frequent QC testing verifies the integrity of the testing device, testing supplies and confirms that the test is performing properly for each patient test. QC testing also may be indicated after POCT device maintenance, any time a POCT device has been dropped, or if patient results do not match the patient symptoms.

Documentation of QC testing is required. Some POCT devices can capture this information electronically, and other methods require manual documentation. When interpreting the QC result, it is imperative to verify that the controls performed as expected. Any time a QC result does not perform as expected (the results are not within the predetermined range), no further patient testing should be performed until the QC error is corrected. The test procedure should provide guidance to resolve the error. Additional guidance can be obtained from the test manufacturer. Documentation of successful QC performance is required to confirm that the test system was able to produce valid test results on the same day that patient testing was performed (**Fig. 7–3**).

TECHNICAL TIP

Patient test results can never be reported if the QC test results are not in range. The problem must be resolved and the test repeated.

URINE DIPSTICK QUALITY CONTROL LOG
for
Chemstrip 10

Quality Control **Level 2 (Abnormal)** Lot # __44461__   Quality Control Exp. Date __04/30/09__

Reagent lot # _____   Reagent Exp. Date _____

Date	Sp. Gravity	pH	Leuko	Nitrite	Protein	Glucose	Ketones	Urobil	Bilirubin	Blood	Tech
QC Range	1.000–1.015	7–9	Tr–2+	Pos	30–500 (1+–3+)	100–1000	1+–3+	Pos	1+–3+	Tr–250 (tr–3+)	

POCT-5   **Reviewed** _____

FIGURE 7–3. Example of urine dipstick QC log for Chemstrip 10 (abnormal control).

Procedures

CLIA requires that operators performing POCT follow manufacturers' guidelines and that written test procedures must be available to all testing personnel. It is important to understand that POCT procedures vary among manufacturers; therefore, package inserts and procedures in the procedure manual are not interchangeable. The procedure manual must be updated when a facility changes to a different manufacturer. Testing personnel must read the entire package insert or procedure manual before performing the test.

> **TECHNICAL TIP**
> Written test procedures must be available to all testing personnel.

The information in package inserts includes the specimen collection and handling, safety precautions, instrument maintenance and calibration, reagent storage requirements, procedural steps, interpretation of results and normal values, and sources of error. Manufacturers also provide training materials and assistance in troubleshooting technical problems.

> **TECHNICAL TIP**
> Recorded results must be legible, in a location where they may be reviewed by the health-care provider and easily retrieved when needed.

Areas in which POCT is performed are required to maintain a procedure manual that is readily available to all testing personnel. The procedure manual contains the information provided in the package inserts from the instrumentation, reagents, and controls for each procedure, the purpose of the test, and identifies who may perform the test. It also contains site-specific information, such as the location of supplies, special handling requirements, patient identification procedures for devices with connectivity, instructions for reporting and recording results, and the protocol to follow when critically low or high test results are encountered.

All patient test results must be recorded in the patient's permanent medical record. The patient test result must include the patient name and identification number, the initials of the operator who performed the test, the date the test was performed, and the facility where the test was performed. In many cases, the hospital computer system will capture this information when patient test results are entered.

Common POCT Errors

One statistic of interest is that laboratory test results influence approximately 70 percent of medical decisions. A common misconception is that POCT can be performed with minimal or no training since many POCTs are only screening tests and the techniques to perform a test are usually quite simple. It is important to understand that whether tests are only for screening, or used to monitor ongoing therapy, they have value. If the test was of no value, it would not be needed. Each result has the potential to shape a patient's outcome in a positive or negative way, and incorrect results can negatively affect patient care, treatment, and outcome. The following scenario illustrates examples of possible negative outcomes for a qualitative urine dipstick test to identify blood in urine.

Preanalytic failure: Failure to obtain the specimen from the correct patient and/or failure to label the specimen with the correct patient name would mean that the right results would be charted on the wrong patient. Failure to collect the specimen in a clean container may cause a false-positive test since bleach residue can cause a false-positive result.

Analytic failure: Failure to perform QC could cause a wrong result if the test strips had been compromised since the test strip integrity was not verified. Failure to read the test strip at the correct time by interpreting the result too early could result in the difference between a negative or positive screening result.

Postanalytic failure: Failure to document the result in the medical record may result in questioning the medical necessity of a confirmatory test. A result that drives a treatment plan must be recorded in the permanent medical record.

All incorrect results can affect the patient outcome by influencing the way the patient is treated, or not treated, and the sequence of ordering additional diagnostic tests based on that simple screening test. **Table 7–2** lists the common errors associated with POCT.

Critical Elements: The Magnificent Seven

Each time a POCT is performed, there are multiple opportunities to make an error that could result in a negative patient outcome. It is impossible to list all of the sources of error and the resulting outcome for the ever growing list of POCTs. Listed below are the critical elements for good laboratory practice that when followed, will prevent the majority of common POCT errors.

1. Patient identification—Identify the correct patient. Use the full name and a second identifier on all samples, requisitions, and reports.
2. Proper specimen collection—Ensure the correct sample type is collected, use correct collection technique, label all specimens, and handle and transport specimens according to procedure.
3. Proper storage of testing supplies—Store reagents at the correct storage temperature and never use an expired test reagent or collection device.
4. QC—Always perform and document QC as required and confirm that QC results are within the expected range before any patient testing is performed.
5. Sample application and test performance—Always follow manufacturers' instructions for applying the sample to the test device and strictly follow test-timing instructions.
6. Result interpretation—Refer to the test procedure for correct interpretation of test result, confirmatory testing that may be required, and guidance for identification and communication of critical results.
7. Documentation of results—Results must be recorded in the permanent medical record, legible, and easily retrieved.

Safety

As health-care professionals, patient safety and the safety of the POCT operator is the responsibility of the POCT operator. Blood and body fluid precautions must be followed for each test procedure. Since POCT may be performed directly at the patient's bedside, care also must be taken to identify and reduce the risk for a POCT device to spread infection between patients. Use of gloves, personal protective equipment, hand washing, and POCT device cleaning maintenance must be strictly followed. As a rule, reusable, spring-loaded lancing devices used in home-care settings are not suitable for institutional use since they have been documented to transmit hepatitis between patients. Additionally, care must be taken to protect patients, staff, and POCT devices in both protective and infection isolation environments.

Regulatory Compliance

All laboratory testing is regulated by the federal law CLIA '88 (Clinical Laboratory Improvement Act of 1988) and is enforced by the Centers for Medicare & Medicaid Services (CMS). CLIA defines the standards and guidelines for performing POCT and all other laboratory testing. Accrediting organizations, such as the College of American Pathologists (CAP), The Joint Commission (JC) (previously named JCAHO), and the Commission on Laboratory Accreditation (COLA) must follow the minimum requirements for laboratory practice required

TABLE 7–2. Common Errors Associated With POCT

TESTS	ERRORS
Hemoglobin	Failure to adequately fill the cuvette
	Bubbles in the cuvette
Glucose	Use of compromised or expired reagent strips
	Failure to adequately cleanse and dry the capillary puncture site
	Failure to adequately or correctly apply specimen to testing area
	Failure to run controls and document results as required
iSTAT Profiles	Failure to identify the patient correctly in the meter
	Failure to observe cartridge warm-up time
	Failure to comply with room temperature expiration dates
	Returning room temperature cartridges to refrigerated storage
	Underfilled or overfilled cartridges
	Squeezing the cartridge when closing
	Moving the device while analyzing a specimen
	Failure to upload meter for timely data transfer
Urinalysis	Use of compromised or expired reagent strips
	Incorrect reaction timing
	Leaving reagent strips in the specimen too long
Occult Blood (guaiac slide methods)	Failure to use the correct sample type for the test kit
	Failure to apply the correct amount of sample on the slide
	Failure to wait specified time after sample is applied to add the developer reagent
	Patients not given pre-collection instructions
Toxicology Profile	Use of incorrectly stored or expired kits
	Misinterpretation of patient and control results
Group A Streptococcus	Using cotton or calcium alginate collection swabs
	Use of compromised or expired reagent kits
	Failure to observe the internal control
	Incorrect collection or timing
Urine Pregnancy Test	Failure to test a first morning specimen
	Addition of reagents in the wrong order
	Misinterpretation of test and control results
Immunoassay Kits	Using reagents from different kits
	Failure to follow the step-by-step instructions
	Use of incorrectly stored or expired kits
	Misinterpretation of test and control results
	Failure to observe and document internal control results
POC Meters (analyzers) with Data Management	Failure to identify the patient correctly in the meter
	Failure to follow correct timing for application of sample to test strip/test cartridge
	Failure to follow correct timing for placing test strip/test cartridge in the meter
	Failure to upload meter for timely data transfer
Coagulation Tests	Failure to adequately cleanse and dry the capillary puncture site
	Failure to follow manufacturer's instructions for specimen collection
	Prematurely performing the capillary puncture before test strip/test cartridge is ready to accept the sample
	Inadequate application of sample

by CLIA. Accrediting organization standards customarily have more stringent regulatory requirements than CLIA. It is important to understand that the regulations, however ominous they may seem, are in place to provide a minimum standard of quality for all laboratory testing. Compliance with CLIA and accrediting organizations' regulatory standards is mandatory and is normally evaluated using a biannual inspection process. Failure to comply with the regulatory standards can lead to federal sanctions, loss of accreditation and the ability to legally perform all laboratory testing.

Laboratory testing is classified into four complexity categories: waived, moderate complexity, high complexity, and provider performed microscopy procedures (PPMP). Most POCT is waived, moderate complexity, or PPMP. The complexity is assigned by the U.S. Food and Drug Administration (FDA) and is based on the skill level required to perform the test. Waived testing does not have any personnel education requirements. Moderate complexity testing requires that testing personnel have a minimum of a high school diploma or equivalent. PPMP testing may only be performed by licensed providers, such as physicians, nurse practitioners, physician assistants, and midwives, etc. High-complexity testing requires operators with specific laboratory science education, or also can be performed by staff that meets the moderate complexity requirements provided the testing is directly supervised by a laboratory professional.

Training and Competency Assessment

All POCT operators must receive training prior to performing patient testing. Competency assessment ensures testing procedures are performed consistently and accurately. Training and competency assessment must encompass the three phases of testing. Competency can be evaluated by methods, such as observation, evaluating adequacy of documentation, or blind test of samples with known values, such as QC materials, proficiency testing samples, or previously analyzed patient samples, and written quizzes. Competency assessment is required by CLIA regulations for all POCT operators who perform moderate and high complexity testing at 6 months and 1 year after initial training. After the first year, competency must be assessed and validated annually. Most accrediting agencies also require annual competency assessment for staff performing waived tests.

POCT Future

The future of POCT will be driven by the increased demand for rapid testing and a broader scope of clinically relevant information. POC device technology will continue to develop portable, stand-alone devices with diverse test menus. Robust data management and connectivity to the patient electronic medical record will become the standard of care. New therapies also will force the evolution of new tests and test methods including noninvasive and alternate sample technologies. Healthcare, in general, is a dynamic profession and change in this field is constant. POCT will continue to play an increasing role in providing quality results in diverse patient care environments.

Point-Of-Care Exercise

1. A POCT operator performs daily bedside glucose tests on an inpatient using a POCT glucose meter. Daily results for the patient were:

   Day 1—100 mg/dL
   Day 2—105 mg/dL
   Day 3—98 mg/dL
   Today the POC operator gets a result of 48 mg/dL. The patient states no change in diet or routine in the past 24 hours.

   a. What should the POCT operator do?

   _____

   _____

   b. What three things could be a cause of an incorrect glucose value?
   1. _____
   2. _____
   3. _____

2. A POCT operator performed the daily morning QC on the glucose meter. The results were:

   Abnormal low = 50 mg/dL
   Abnormal high = 200 mg/dL
   The range for the abnormal low is 33 to 57 mg/dL; the abnormal high range is 278 to 418 mg/dL.

   a. Can the POCT operator report patient results?

   _____

   b. What actions are required by the POCT operator?

   _____

   c. What is a possible cause of any discrepancy?

   _____

REVIEW QUESTIONS

1. Preanalytical errors in POCT include all of the following EXCEPT:
   a. Improper storage of test materials
   b. Failure to check reagent expiration dates
   c. Performing the test too near the patient
   d. Performing the test on the wrong patient

2. QC is part of the:
   a. Preanalytical phase
   b. Analytical phase
   c. Postanalytical phase
   d. Collection phase

3. Test result documentation is part of the:
   a. Preanalytical phase
   b. Analytical phase
   c. Laboratory phase
   d. Postanalytical phase

4. QC of POCT should be performed by:
   a. The POCT supervisor
   b. The person performing patient testing
   c. A POCT performer and a supervisor
   d. A medical technologist

5. Acceptable QC can ensure all of the following EXCEPT:
   a. Correct patient identification
   b. Integrity of the testing materials
   c. Correct performance of the test
   d. Correct functioning of the testing device

6. The two levels of control samples that must be tested to ensure test result accuracy are:
   a. Baseline and elevated
   b. Normal and abnormal
   c. Acceptable and nonacceptable
   d. Internal and proficiency

7. To determine the proper maintenance of a POCT instrument, the operator should:
   a. Attend a proficiency class
   b. Read the package insert
   c. Contact the manufacturer
   d. Consult with another caregiver

8. When performing POCT, a caregiver must be sure to document results of:
   a. Patient tests
   b. Quality control
   c. Electronic controls
   d. All of the above

9. The recommended specimen for urine pregnancy testing is a:
   a. Random specimen
   b. First morning specimen
   c. Midstream clean-catch specimen
   d. Timed specimen

10. Six months after beginning employment a health-care worker is given a sample by the POCT supervisor and asked to perform a screening test for Group A Streptococcus and return the results to the supervisor. The employee is performing:
    a. QC
    b. Compliance testing
    c. Patient testing
    d. Competency testing

Internet Help

www.cms.hhs.gov/CLIA/
wwwn.cdc.gov/dls/
   bestpractices/
www.cdc.gov/clia/
www.accessdata.fda.gov/
   scripts/cdrh/cfdocs/
   cfCLIA/search.cfm

www.osha.gov/SLTC/etools/hospital/
   lab/lab.html#OSHA_Laboratory
   _Standard

8

Intravenous Insertion and Central Venous Catheter Access

LEARNING OBJECTIVES

Upon completion of this unit, the reader will be able to:

- State the proper patient identification procedures.
- Describe the communication skills required for assessing the level of patient comprehension of the procedure.
- Describe the infection-control guidelines and standards associated with the equipment and procedures performed according to the Centers for Disease Control and Prevention (CDC) guidelines and those of your facility.
- Discuss the proper selection and use of equipment necessary for insertion and maintenance of an IV catheter.
- Discuss the adequate preparation of patient.

- Explain the adequate preparation of the venous access site and proper connection of the IV fluids to the catheter.
- Discuss the collection of blood specimens after insertion of an IV catheter.
- Identify and recognize the types of central venous catheters (CVCs).
- Explain how to safely draw blood through the CVC and obtain the proper specimens for laboratory testing.
- Identify the correct methods of infection-control techniques used when manipulating a CVC.

Introduction

Advances in the delivery of medications have produced an increase in patients receiving direct venous infusion of medications. These changes have resulted in the need to use additional methods for the collection of blood specimens.

The purpose of this unit is to familiarize you with the collection of blood via insertion of a peripheral IV catheter or via a CVC while it remains in the patient. The variety of these central venous access devices (CVADs) also has produced a variety of different procedures required to collect a quality blood specimen while maintaining the integrity of the catheter.

Peripheral Access Devices

Introduction

Peripheral access devices, including peripheral IV lines and midline peripheral catheters, are commonly used in hospitals and clinics to administer medications and IV fluids. The abbreviation IV means intravenous, or the giving of fluids directly into the circulatory system by way of a catheter.

The peripheral IV insertion procedure is performed under aseptic technique, using a selected IV catheter that is inserted through the skin into a vein. IV catheters come in a variety of sizes ranging from 14-gauge to 24-gauge, the smaller the gauge number, the larger the catheter size. It is recommended to choose the smallest size and shortest length to accommodate the prescribed therapy. In an emergency situation, a larger catheter size may be used, such as a 16- or 18-gauge. The most common, all purpose IV catheter size is a 20-gauge. It is essential for health-care providers to understand the techniques and be proficient in obtaining and maintaining IV access for continuum of care of their patients.

The midline peripheral catheter is inserted into the arm near the inside of the elbow and threaded up inside the large vein approximately 6 inches. These catheters are inserted by specially trained health-care professionals. Midline catheters last approximately 6 weeks and are ideal for some short-term antibiotic therapy.

Unlike the procedures for blood collection from CVCs, blood for laboratory testing is only drawn from peripheral access devices at the time of their insertion.

Peripheral IV Insertion Procedure

1. Introduce yourself and explain the procedure. Allow the patient the opportunity to ask questions and to verbalize understanding.
2. Wash your hands, apply gloves, and prepare the equipment needed for insertion.
3. Follow proper identification procedure to identify the patient for whom the order was written.
4. Choose the appropriate size catheter.
5. Collect the necessary supplies and equipment, such as:

   - A tourniquet (single use/latex-free)
   - Chlorhexidine gluconate sponge
   - Betadine and alcohol pads (optional)
   - A 10-mL saline flush syringe
   - A one-way valve connector device
   - An occlusive dressing
   - Tape—2 to 3, ¼-inch strips
   - 2×2 gauze pads

6. Verify what type of IV fluid is to be given. Follow strict hand-washing guidelines and maintain sterile technique throughout the process.
7. Fill the drip chamber and examine the IV bag and tubing for leaks. Verify the IV tubing is free of any air bubbles, and clamp off the tubing.
8. Remove gloves and wash hands. Apply new gloves.
9. Connect the saline flush syringe to the one-way valve connector device and flush with 1 mL of solution. Leave the end cap on the connector device to maintain sterility. It may be helpful to place a disposable pad down first on the work surface, to help keep equipment and supplies clean and organized.
10. To position the patient, hyperextend the patient's arm and place an absorbent pad or towel under the arm to prevent soiling of the bed linen.

11. Apply the tourniquet about 3 to 4 inches above the puncture site. Palpate the vein to determine its location and direction.

12. Scrub site vigorously with a chlorhexidine gluconate sponge for 30 seconds to sterilize site. Alternately, the site can be wiped with an alcohol pad in a circular motion, followed by a Betadine swab. Start in a circular motion, from the puncture site working outward approximately 1½ to 2 inches. Allow Betadine to dry.

13. Remove the catheter from the package, inspect quickly for any defect on the outside of the catheter. Anchor the vein with nondominant hand, and grasp catheter firmly between the thumb and index finger of the dominant hand with bevel of the needle inside the catheter pointed up at a 15- to 30-degree angle.

14. Insert the tip of the catheter into the vein, observing for a flashback of blood into the small chamber of the catheter. Once a flashback is observed start advancing the catheter using the thumb while holding the catheter in place with the index finger. Some health-care professionals use a two-handed technique, by advancing with one hand, while the other hand holds the catheter in place. The catheter will advance easier when the vein remains anchored and skin traction is maintained. Both methods are considered adequate for successful insertion.

15. When the catheter is inserted into the vein, remove the tourniquet. Remove the needle device by gently twisting to unscrew the needle device from the catheter while applying light pressure to the top of the catheter. Connect the one-way connector with the flush syringe or blood collection syringe attached.

TECHNICAL TIP

When pulling back on the syringe, does the blood flow back easily? Is it easy to flush back into vein?

SAFETY TIP

It is very important to secure IV tubing to the patient, and explain precautions related to unassisted ambulation to the patient.

16. If laboratory tests are not ordered, flush with 2 to 3 mL of saline solution and pull back to check blood return. Blood collection from a peripheral IV is discussed in the following section.

17. While flushing, observe for any signs of swelling in the area or any pain the patient may be experiencing.

18. Once adequate blood flow and flushing has been established, secure the device with tape, over and around the catheter. Place a sterile occlusive dressing to cover entire insertion site.

19. Attach the necessary IV fluids to the device, open clamps, and run fluids as ordered.

20. Label the occlusive dressing with the date, time, catheter size, and initials.

21. Follow institutional policies regarding maintenance.

22. Dispose of all sharps into an approved sharps container. Other materials can be placed into the nonbiohazard waste container.

23. Remove gloves and wash hands.

24. The IV site should be inspected daily for any signs of redness, drainage, and swelling.

Blood Collection From Peripheral Vascular Access Devices (Peripheral IVs and Midline Catheters)

Blood specimen collection from a peripheral vascular access device is performed only at the time of initial insertion of the device. Do not routinely collect blood specimens from indwelling peripheral or midline catheters. At the time of insertion blood may be collected prior to administration of treatment. Refer to step 15 under "Peripheral IV Insertion Procedure," in preceding text.

Blood can be collected by attaching an appropriate size syringe or syringes to the catheter connector and slowly withdrawing the required amount of blood. The blood is then transferred to the required evacuated tubes using a blood transfer device. Attaching a needle to the syringe and puncturing the evacuated tube stopper not only is dangerous to the collector but also may result in hemolysis of the specimen.

Blood from the catheter connector also can be collected directly into evacuated tubes using the following procedure.

1. Attach blunt cannula of tube holder into catheter adapter.
2. Advance specimen tube onto stopper puncturing needle in the holder.
3. Observe for flow of blood into the tube.
4. Allow tube to fill.
5. If more than one tube of blood is needed, change tubes slowly and steadily, taking care not to move catheter in cannulated vein and cause the patient undue pain or discomfort.
6. Mix tubes as they are removed from the holder.
7. Remove holder and continue with the original procedure.

Blood Collection From Central Venous Catheters

Introduction

CVCs are a special type of catheter that is inserted by a physician or a certified health-care professional as either an internal catheter or external catheter into a large vessel of the body. CVCs are used when an individual requires long-term medication administration (antibiotics or chemotherapy) or nutritional support. CVCs also are considered when the patient's vasculature prohibits placing a peripheral IV and frequent blood draws are warranted. The choice of what type and whether it is an internal or external catheter depends on the specific need and preference of the health-care professional inserting the catheter.

Types

There are four types of CVCs: (1) nontunneled, noncuffed; (2) tunneled; (3) implanted; and (4) peripherally inserted central catheter (PICC).

NONTUNNELED, NONCUFFED CENTRAL CATHETER

This type of catheter is inserted directly through the skin and into a large vein in the jugular, subclavian, or femoral veins. They are commonly called triple-lumen catheters, having one to three ports to access with antireflux valve connector end caps on the ends of ports. They are covered with an occlusive waterproof dressing.

TUNNELED

Broviac, Hickman, and Groshong are examples of external catheters, meaning that part of the catheter is on the outside of the body, with the tip of the catheter placed internally in a large vein just above the heart. These require a sterile dressing to be applied over their insertion site.

IMPLANTED PORT

This implanted catheter is placed under the skin surgically by a physician, usually at the collarbone. It consists of a self-sealing septum housed in a metal or plastic case. The catheter is threaded into the superior vena cava (SVC). The port is palpated to locate the septum, and is accessed with a specially designed noncoring needle, often called a Huber needle. This needle has a deflected tip and is configured at a 90-degree angle. This type of port may be a single- or double-lumen catheter. It is commonly used in long-term drug therapies, such as the administration of chemotherapy but also can be used for blood draws (**Fig. 8–1**).

PERIPHERALLY INSERTED CENTRAL CATHETERS (PICC LINES)

This type of catheter is inserted through a large peripheral vein into the lower one third of the superior vena cava (SVC) to the junction of the SVC in the right atrium (SVC/RA). Specially trained health-care professionals insert the catheter by threading the catheter through an introducer needle with about 6 to 10 inches of catheter exposed and covered by an occlusive dressing. There is an antireflux valve connector device attached to the end of the catheter, where the IV is connected or blood specimens are removed. This catheter can be left in for several weeks to months.

TECHNICAL TIP

Flushing peripheral IVs and CVCs is performed to ensure and maintain patency of the catheter, and to prevent mixing of medications and solutions that are incompatible. Follow manufacturers' instructions for correct use and institutional policy and procedure for flushing.

Blood Specimen Collection

Blood specimen collection for laboratory testing, donor collection, or therapeutic indications can be routinely drawn from certain central vascular access devices. Blood specimens may not be drawn from an infusion administration set or proximal to an existing infusion site. It is necessary that the blood collector is knowledgeable about blood collection and the correct order of draw. Refer to the laboratory for confirmation of order of draw and appropriate collection equipment.

Patient Assessment and Education

1. Obtain and review health-care provider's order.
2. Verify patient's identity using two independent identifiers, not including patient's room number.
3. Provide patient with information on blood collection procedure.
4. Obtain patient's consent.
5. Place patient in recumbent position, as tolerated.
6. Assess patient.

FIGURE 8–1. Implanted port.

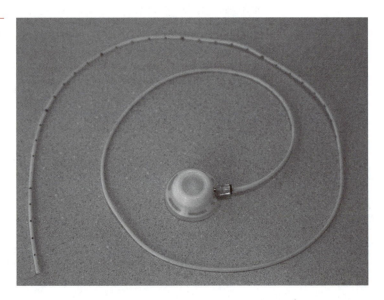

Collection of Blood From Central Venous Lines

Equipment

Two pairs of sterile gloves
Alcohol wipes or chlorhexidine gluconate sponge
Betadine wipes (optional)
2—10-mL syringes filled with normal saline, for flush
2—5-mL syringes
Blood collection tubes for ordered tests
Evacuated tube holder
1 (10- or 20-mL) syringe for blood collection
Blood transfer device
1 to 2 (5-mL) syringe(s) filled with heparinized saline, for flushing after using the saline flush.
   (Optional) Refer to your facility's policy regarding the use of heparin flush solutions in central lines.

General Procedure

1. Collect the above materials and place them on a flat work surface within easy reach, such as a bedside table or rolling tray table covered with a disposable pad.
2. Proper hand washing should be followed, especially when manipulating a central line catheter as most catheters are placed into large vasculature in and around the heart.
3. Apply gloves and prepare equipment, identify the patient, explain procedure, and allow for questions.
4. Position the patient in a supine position. Have the patient turn his or her head away from the direction or position of the catheter.
5. Position the equipment within a reachable distance, remove gloves, wash hands, and apply mask and sterile gloves.
6. When collecting blood from CVADs, it is essential that an amount of blood equal to 1.5 to 2 times the fill volume of the CVAD be discarded or conserved prior to collecting the test specimen. This is to avoid contamination of the specimen with infusion or flush material.

Procedures for the various types of central line catheters vary slightly and will be discussed separately.

Nontunneled, Noncuffed Central Catheter

PROCEDURE

1. These catheters can be single-, double-, or triple-lumen catheters. When being used for continuous infusion; the infusion should be placed on hold for several minutes before drawing laboratory specimens (**Fig. 8–2**).
2. A 30-second scrub of the port end with an alcohol pad should take place before drawing laboratory specimens (**Fig. 8–3**).
3. Connect a 5-mL syringe to the access device on the end of the port and discard or conserve 5 mL of blood. If using a triple-lumen catheter, clamp all ports and withdraw from the proximal port of the catheter.
4. Withdraw the required amount based on laboratory tests ordered, using a syringe of appropriate size or evacuated tubes and a holder.
5. Unclamp all ports and flush all ports with saline and resume infusion as ordered.

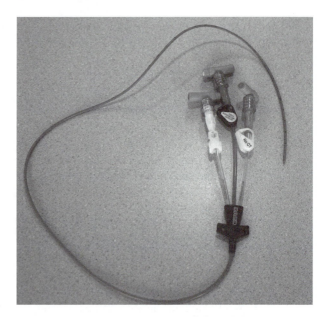

FIGURE 8–2. Triple-lumen catheter.

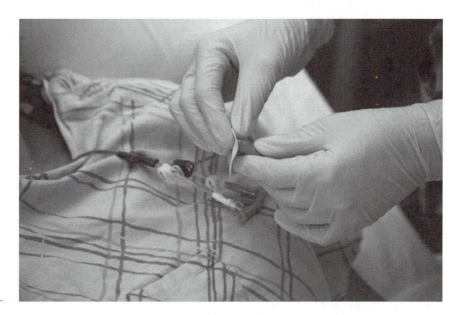

FIGURE 8–3. Cleaning port end of catheter with alcohol.

6. Connect a blood transfer device to the collection syringe and insert evacuated tubes. Allow each tube to fill; do not force blood from collection syringe as this may cause hemolysis of the red blood cells in the sample, and falsely alter certain laboratory analytes.

7. Label each tube appropriately, according to your facility's procedures and place into a biohazard collection bag and send to the laboratory.

8. Clean all used and unused equipment, remove gloves, wash hands, assist in repositioning patient, and thank the patient for his or her cooperation.

Hickman and Groshong Catheters

Hickman catheters may be single- or multilumen. The most common is the double-lumen, which has two color-coded tails; the white port is for routine IV fluids and medications and the red port is for blood draws and infusing blood products.

EQUIPMENT

2–10-mL syringes
Alcohol pads
Evacuated blood tubes
2–10-mL normal saline flush syringes

PROCEDURE

1. Assemble equipment needed, wash hands, and apply gloves and mask.
2. Clean the end cap and rubber septum of the red line by cleansing with a 30-second alcohol scrub.
3. Connect a saline syringe to the line and gently flush line with a small amount of saline, observe for any difficulty flushing the line; then pull back on the plunger of the syringe until blood appears in the line.
4. As the blood appears, flush with remaining amount of saline to clear the line; withdraw 10 or 20 mL of blood and discard or conserve.
5. Change to a new syringe to draw required amount of blood necessary for testing or attach evacuated tube holder. Use a blood transfer device to place blood from the syringe into appropriate evacuated blood collection tubes. Mix tubes 3 to 8 times by gentle inversion.
6. Close clamp on line, apply another flush syringe to the line, unclamp and gently flush in a slow pulsing motion. After line is flushed with saline, some references state to flush with heparin solution and close clamp. Refer to your facility's policy and standards of care protocol for complete guidelines.
7. Remove all syringes and transfer devices and discard all equipment in an appropriate sharps container.
8. Remove gloves, wash hands, and place labels and documentation on tubes. Put laboratory specimens in biohazard specimen bag for transport to the laboratory.

Groshong Catheter

This catheter is a clear silicone external catheter with a blue radiopaque line running alongside the length of the catheter. The Groshong catheter has a three-position valve at the end of the catheter tip. The valve opens to allow blood collection and fluid infusion but does not allow backflow of blood. Therefore, use of heparin is not needed with this type of catheter and is not recommended.

The procedure is very similar to that of the Hickman catheter, with one exception; no heparin is used with this catheter.

PROCEDURE

1. Wash hands and apply gloves and mask.
2. Clean the lumen with a 30-second scrub with an alcohol pad and secure a 10-mL saline syringe to the line. Gently flush with a small amount of saline (2 to 3 mL). Pull back the plunger of the syringe until blood appears, about 2 to 3 mL; then flush the remaining amount of saline back into the line.

3. Using a 10-mL syringe, withdraw 10 mL of blood and discard or conserve it. If samples will be collected for coagulation studies, 20 mL of blood must be discarded.
4. Attach a volume-appropriate syringe to draw the amount of blood needed for collection tubes. Use a blood transfer device when blood is collected by syringe to transfer blood into blood sample tubes and mix 3 to 8 times by gentle inversion.
5. Flush line with 20 mL of sterile saline and clamp.
6. Discard all used equipment, remove mask and gloves, and wash hands.

Implanted Port

This port is surgically placed, under the skin, usually located in the upper chest near the collarbone. This device requires the use of a noncoring or a Huber needle.

EQUIPMENT

Sterile drape, gloves
A noncoring or Huber needle, 1- or 1½-inch length depending on the depth of the implant
2—10-mL syringes
2—10-mL flush syringes filled with saline
1—10-mL syringe filled with heparinized flush solution
Chlorhexidine gluconate sponge or alcohol and Betadine pads
1—5-mL syringe
2 × 2 gauze pads
Dressing to cover insertion site if needle is removed
Luer-Lok adapter

PROCEDURE

1. Assemble equipment.
2. Wash hands and apply gloves and mask.
3. Palpate the shoulder area to locate and identify the septum of the access port.
4. Prep the area with a vigorous scrub using a chlorhexidine gluconate applicator. If using alcohol and Betadine wipes, prep a circular motion from within to outward, approximately 4 to 6 inches, allow solution to dry completely.
5. Connect the Huber needle tubing on the end of one 10-mL saline flush syringe and prime the needle with saline until it is expelled.
6. Locate the septum of the port with the nondominant hand, firmly anchor the port between the thumb and the forefinger.
7. Holding the Huber needle with the other hand, puncture the skin and insert the needle at a 90-degree angle into the septum using firm pressure. Advance the needle until resistance is met and the needle touches the back wall of the port.
8. Inject 1 to 2 mL of saline, observe the area for swelling and ease of flow; if swelling occurs, reposition the needle in the port without withdrawing it from the skin. If there is no swelling, aspirate for blood return. If blood return is observed, continue to flush with saline.
9. Using the same syringe, aspirate 10 mL of blood and discard or conserve it. If samples will be collected for coagulation studies, discard 20 mL.
10. Attach the Luer-Lok adapter of the syringe or the evacuated tube holder to the needle tubing and collect the blood necessary for ordered laboratory tests. Dispense the blood into the appropriate blood sample tubes using a blood transfer device if a syringe is used. Mix the blood by gentle inversion 3 to 8 times.

11. Flush the needle and the port with 10 mL of saline.
12. Change syringes and flush with 3 mL of heparinized saline or according to your facility's policy.
13. Remove the needle and apply a sterile dressing over site.
14. Label specimens appropriately, remove gloves, wash hands, and send specimens to laboratory for testing.

Peripherally Inserted Central Catheters

To obtain blood from a PICC, the catheter size must be 4 French (Fr) or greater in size. If a PICC is being used for total parental nutrition (TPN), it cannot be used for blood drawing. It also is important not to apply a tourniquet or a blood pressure cuff to the arm with the PICC line, since this may occlude or collapse the catheter.

PROCEDURE

1. Wash hands and apply gloves before any manipulation to the catheter takes place.
2. If there is an infusion in progress, the infusion should be placed on hold. Cleanse the injection port with a 30-second scrub of alcohol, flush the catheter with 10 mL of sterile saline; then gently aspirate a 5-mL waste and discard.
3. Using a volume-appropriate syringe, slowly and gently withdraw the needed amount of blood for required laboratory tests. If any difficulty aspirating from the catheter is experienced, try repositioning the patient's arm by flexion or extension or elevation above the patient's head. Attempt to flush the catheter and aspirate again.
4. After obtaining the samples needed, use a 10-mL or larger syringe to flush the catheter. Use a pulsed type motion while flushing with the saline and follow with 2 mL of heparin flush solution if not resuming the IV fluids.
5. PICC line catheters require frequent observations. Assessing insertion site and changing of dressing and injection cap are necessary to avoid infection. Check with your facility's policy regarding manipulation or use of PICC lines.

> **TECHNICAL TIP**
>
> Proficiency in the care of catheters will result with continued practice of technique and skills.

Blood Conservation

Reinfusion of blood (instead of wasting blood) from CVADs for laboratory draws is an alternative procedure for patients in hospitals on the Blood Conservation Program. This procedure uses a three-way stopcock device with a sterile syringe attached, to reinfuse the blood/saline back to the patient.

PROCEDURE

1. Discontinue administration of all infusates into the CVAD (all lumens) prior to obtaining blood samples. If the lumen to be used for laboratory draws has an infusion, cap the tubing with a male/female cap when disconnecting.
2. When drawing from multilumen catheters, the proximal lumen is the preferred lumen from which to obtain the specimen. Use clamp on lumen to control blood flow and to help eliminate confusion with the stopcock.
3. Attach a 10-mL prefilled saline syringe to a three-way stopcock. Prime the stopcock with saline (**Fig. 8–4**).
4. Disinfect injection cap with alcohol wipe using vigorous friction scrub on the top and in the grooves for 15 seconds. If the laboratory draw is for a blood culture, scrub the injection cap with an alcohol wipe for 30 seconds.

5. Attach stopcock with syringe to injection cap (**Fig. 8–5**).
6. Unclamp lumen and flush with remainder of saline. If the only lumen available to draw blood has TPN infusing, flush with 18 to 19 mL of saline.
7. Clamp lumen and/or turn stopcock to "off" position to syringe port (**Fig. 8–6**).
8. Remove syringe and apply a new empty syringe to the same stopcock port.
9. Turn stopcock to "off" position to the unaccessed port. Unclamp lumen. Aspirate 5 mL blood into the empty syringe. Leave the syringe attached.
10. Attach another empty syringe to the second stopcock port (**Fig. 8–7**).
11. Turn stopcock to "off" position to the blood-filled syringe.
12. Draw blood specimen into empty syringe or attach an evacuated tube holder to collect blood directly into collection tubes. (**Fig. 8–8**).
13. Turn stopcock "off" to specimen port. Remove specimen.
14. When using a syringe, transfer specimen to evacuated tubes using a blood transfer device.
15. Reinfuse blood from previously filled syringe.
16. Remove stopcock and syringe. Cleanse injection cap with alcohol pad.
17. Attach prefilled saline syringe and flush with 18 to 19 mL of saline (**Fig. 8–9**).
18. Resume all infusions in all lumens.

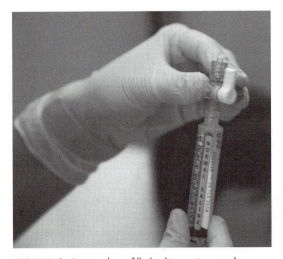

FIGURE 8–4. Attach prefilled saline syringe to three-way stopcock.

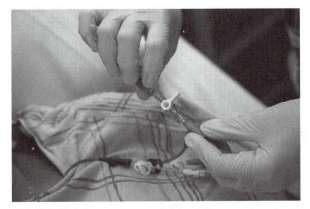

FIGURE 8–5. Stopcock with syringe attached to injection cap.

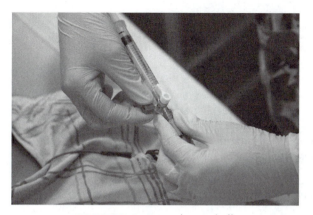

FIGURE 8–6. Stopcock turned off.

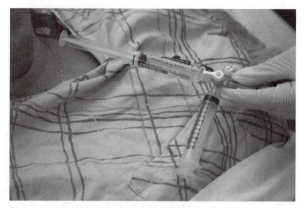

FIGURE 8–7. Attach empty syringe.

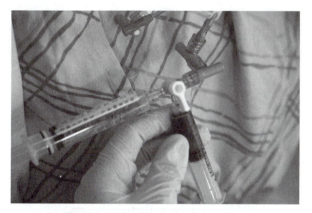

FIGURE 8–8. Blood drawn into empty syringe.

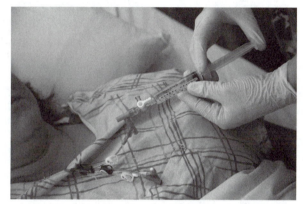

FIGURE 8–9. Flush with saline.

Intravenous and CVCs Exercise

1. A new hospital employee at a hospital that has adopted the Blood Conservation Program is rechecking the procedure as she prepares her equipment prior to collecting blood for a complete blood count (CBC).
   a. How many syringes will she need if she is collecting the blood using a syringe?
   b. How many syringes will she need if she is using the evacuated tube system?
   c. What additional piece of equipment will she need beside the collection tubes when using the evacuated tube system?

2. State two ways in which blood collected after insertion of a peripheral IV could be hemolyzed.

3. A student asks you to explain the following terms and their purpose:
   a. Flashback
   b. Flush syringes

Peripheral IV Insertion Evaluation

Rating System   **2 = Satisfactorily**   **1 = Needs Improvement**   **0 = Incorrect/Did Not Perform**

NAME:_____

Prior to entering patient's room:

_____ **1.** Checks IV fluid for correct name, expiration date, contamination, and leaks.

_____ **2.** Spikes bag.

_____ **3.** Fills drip chamber and primes tubing (free of air bubbles).

Enters patient's room:

_____ **4.** Introduces self, establishes rapport.

_____ **5.** Identifies patient.

_____ **6.** Assesses patient history (specifically for allergies).

_____ **7.** Explains procedure to patient.

_____ **8.** Prepares the environment: privacy, lighting, and bed adjustment.

_____ **9.** Prepares equipment.

_____ **10.** Washes hands and dons gloves.

_____ **11.** Applies tourniquet 3–4 inches above puncture site.

_____ **12.** Palpates for suitable vein, releases tourniquet.

_____ **13.** Cleanses puncture site appropriately.

_____ **14.** Reties tourniquet.

_____ **15.** Stabilizes vein and inserts IV catheter watching for flashback.

_____ **16.** Releases tourniquet.

_____ **17.** Advances catheter into vein.

_____ **18.** Occludes vein proximal to catheter.

_____ **19.** Removes needle and disposes of it into proper container.

_____ **20.** Attaches IV tubing to catheter.

_____ **21.** Opens clamp, runs IV to ensure patent line, watches for signs of infiltration.

_____ **22.** Adjusts clamp for correct IV flow per situation.

_____ **23.** Applies sterile dressing to IV site.

_____ **24.** Secures IV with tape or other device.

_____ **25.** Explains precautions and ambulation procedure to patient.

_____ **26.** Maintains aseptic technique and adheres to standard precautions throughout procedure.

Total Points _____
Maximum points 52
COMMENTS

REVIEW QUESTIONS

1. When collecting blood specimens after inserting a peripheral IV catheter the:
   a. Line should be flushed before the blood is collected
   b. Line should be flushed after the blood is collected
   c. Catheter tubing should be taped to the patient first
   d. Tourniquet should not be removed

2. Which of the following is a tunneled catheter?
   a. Midline peripheral catheter
   b. PICC line
   c. Hickman
   d. Peripheral IV

3. Blood collected from CVCs is collected in evacuated tubes by attaching a/an:
   a. Sterile 20-gauge needle to the collection syringe
   b. Evacuated tube holder to the catheter line
   c. Blood transfer device to the collection syringe
   d. Luer-Lok to the catheter line

4. Evacuated tubes containing blood collected from a CVC should be gently mixed:
   a. After the line has been flushed
   b. As soon as they are filled
   c. After they are labeled
   d. As soon as the port has been heparinized

5. Blood can NOT be drawn from which of the following catheters?
   a. Midline peripheral
   b. Groshong
   c. PICC line
   d. Hickman

6. What should the blood collector observe when flushing the IV tubing?
   a. Swelling or pain in the area
   b. Ease of injecting flush solution into the catheter
   c. Ability to obtain blood back into the flush syringe
   d. All of the above

7. Blood can NOT be drawn from a PICC line that is infusing:
   a. Antibiotics
   b. Total parental nutrition
   c. Dextrose
   d. Pain medication

8. A tourniquet should not be applied when collecting blood using:
   a. A peripheral IV catheter
   b. Hickman catheter
   c. PICC line
   d. Implanted port

9. Blood collected from which of the following catheters does not require a waste/conservation tube?
   a. Peripheral IV line
   b. PICC line
   c. Groshong
   d. Hickman

10. Central venous catheters are inserted primarily by:
    a. Physicians
    b. Radiologists
    c. Phlebotomists
    d. Respiratory therapists

Internet Help

Seattle treatment education project. The body. Available at http: // www.thebody.com/content/art1786.html?ts=pf Accessed 8/30/2008.

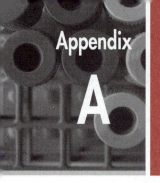
Common Laboratory Tests and the Required Types of Anticoagulants and Volume of Blood Required

TEST	COLLECTION TUBE	MINIMUM AMOUNT	COMMENTS	DEPT.	ABBREVIATION
Ammonia	Lavender	3 mL	Send on ice slurry	C	NH^3
Amylase	Green PST; SST (gel-barrier tube)	3 mL		C	
Antibiotic assay (Gentamicin, tobramycin, vancomycin)	Red (no gel barrier); Clear nongel Microtainer	5 mL	No SST tubes	C	Gent, Tob, Vanco
Antibody ID/Screen	Lavender	7 mL	Blood bank ID	BB	
Beta HCG/Quant.	Green PST; SST	3 mL		C	
Bilirubin	Green PST; SST; Amber Microtainer	1.5 mL	Protect from light	C	Bili
Vitamin B_{12}	Green PST; SST; Red	3 mL		C	
Complete Blood Count	Lavender	3 mL		H	CBC
Cortisol	SST; Red	2 mL	Serum only; Timed specimen	C	
Crossmatch	Lavender; Pink	7 mL	Blood bank ID remains on 72 hours	BB	
D-Dimer	Light blue	4.5 mL	Tube must be full (stable for 4 hours)	CO	D-DI
Ethanol/Alcohol	Gray; Red	3 mL	Do not open tube until testing; may require chain of custody	C	ETOH
Fibrinogen	Light blue	4.5 mL	Tube must be full	CO	
Folate	SST	3 mL		C	
Glucose	Green PST; SST; Red; Gray	3 mL		C	FBS
Hemoglobin/ hematocrit	Lavender	3 mL		H	H&H; Hgb/Hct
Hepatitis panels	SST; Red	6 mL		C	
Ionized calcium	SST; Red; Arterial blood gas syringe	7 mL	Tube must be full; may use arterial blood gas syringe	C	iCA^{2+}
Lactate (Lactic acid)	Green PST; Arterial blood gas syringe	5 mL	Send in ice; analyze in 15 minutes. Draw without tourniquet	C	Lact

TEST	COLLECTION TUBE	MINIMUM AMOUNT	COMMENTS	DEPT.	ABBREVIATION
Lead	Royal blue EDTA; Tan EDTA	2 mL		C	Pb
Lipase	Green PST; SST; Red	3 mL		C	
Lithium	SST; Red	5 mL	Draw 12 hours post dose	C	Li
MI panel (myoglobin, creatine kinase isoenzyme, troponin)	Green PST	3 mL	Stable 4 hours; EDTA plasma from a lavender top tube may be used or a white PPT tube	C	Myo, CK-MB, T
Mononucleosis Screen	SST; Red	3 mL		S	Monotest
pH	Green	3 mL	Send on ice slurry	C	
Platelet	Lavender	3 mL		H	Plt
Prothrombin time	Light blue	4.5 mL	Full tube; stable 24 hours at room temperature	CO	PT
Activated/partial thromboplastin time	Light blue	4.5 mL	Full tube; stable 4 hours refrigerated	CO	PTT/APTT
Protein electrophoresis	SST; Red	3 mL		C	
Reticulocyte count	Lavender	3 mL		H	Retic
Therapeutic drugs (digoxin, theophylline, Phenobarbital, phenytoin, carbamazepine, valproic acid)	Red; Clear non-gel Microtainer	3 mL/(full Microtainer)		Dig, Pheno	Theo, Pheny, Carb, Val Ac
Thyroid-stimulating hormone/Free T4	Green PST; SST	3 mL		C	TSH/T4
Quant proteins (C3, C4, IgG, IgA, IgM, haptoglobin)	SST; Red	3 mL		C	
Sedimentation rate	Lavender	5 mL		H	ESR
Chemistry panels (renal, hepatic, comprehensive, metabolic)	Green PST; SST	3 mL		C	
Lipid panel	Green PST; SST	5 mL		C	HDL, Chol, Trig

This is a list of anticoagulant and specimen requirements for the most common test requests at Methodist Hospital, Omaha, Nebraska, courtesy of Diane Wolff, MT(ASCP), Phlebotomy Supervisor. Each laboratory will have specific test protocols.
Lab department codes: BB = Blood Bank, C = Chemistry, CO = Coagulation, H = Hematology, S = Serology

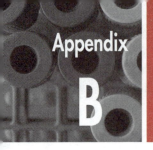

Clinical Correlations of Blood Tests Related to Body Systems

TEST	CLINICAL CORRELATION
CIRCULATORY SYSTEM	
Activated clotting time (ACT)	Heparin therapy
Activated partial thromboplastin time [APTT(PTT)]	Heparin therapy or coagulation disorders
Antibody (Ab) screen	Blood transfusion
Antistreptolysin O (ASO) titer	Rheumatic fever
Antithrombin III	Cardiac risk
Apo-A, Apo-B lipoprotein	Coagulation disorders
Arterial blood gases	Acid/base balance
Aspartate aminotransferase [AST(SGOT)]	Cardiac muscle damage
Bilirubin	Hemolytic disorders
Bleeding time (BT)	Platelet function
Blood culture	Septicemia
Blood group and type	ABO group and Rh factor
Brain natriuretic peptide (BNP)	Congestive heart failure
C-reactive protein (CRP)	Inflammatory disorders
Cholesterol	Coronary artery disease
Complete blood count (CBC)	Anemia, infection, leukemia, or bleeding disorders
Creatine kinase [CK(CPK)]	Myocardial infarction
Creatine kinase isoenzymes (CK-MB)	Myocardial infarction
Disseminated intravascular coagulation (DIC) panel	Coagulation/fibrinolytic systems
Digoxin	Heart stimulant
Direct anti–human globulin test (DAT) or direct Coombs	Anemia or hemolytic disease of the newborn
Erythrocyte sedimentation rate (ESR)	Inflammatory disorders
Fibrin degradation products (FDP)	Disseminated intravascular coagulation
Fibrinogen	Coagulation disorders
Folate	Anemia
Hematocrit (Hct)	Anemia
Hemoglobin (Hgb)	Anemia
Hemoglobin (Hgb) electrophoresis	Hemoglobin abnormalities
High-density lipoprotein (HDL)	Coronary risk
Iron	Anemia
Lactate dehydrogenase [LD(LDH)]	Myocardial infarction
Low-density lipoprotein (LDL)	Coronary risk
Myoglobin	Myocardial infarction
Platelet (Plt) count	Bleeding tendencies
Potassium	Heart contraction/cardiac output
Prothrombin time (PT)	Coumadin therapy and coagulation disorders

CIRCULATORY SYSTEM—cont'd

Reticulocyte (Retic) count	Bone marrow function
Sickle cell screening	Sickle cell anemia
Total iron binding capacity (TIBC)	Anemia
Triglycerides	Coronary artery disease
Troponin I and T	Myocardial infarction
Type and crossmatch (T & C)	Blood transfusion
Type and screen	Blood transfusion
White blood cell (WBC) count	Infections or leukemia
Vitamin B$_{12}$	Anemia

LYMPHATIC SYSTEM

Anti-HIV	Human immunodeficiency virus
Antinuclear antibody (ANA)	Systemic lupus erythematosus/autoimmune disorders
Complete blood count (CBC)	Infectious mononucleosis
Complement levels	Immune system function/autoimmune disorders
Fluorescent antinuclear antibody (FANA)	Systemic lupus erythematosus/autoimmune disorders
Immunoglobulin (Ig) levels	Immune system function
Monospot	Infectious mononucleosis
p24 antigen	Human immunodeficiency virus
Protein electrophoresis	Multiple myeloma
T-cell count	Immune function/HIV monitoring
Viral load	HIV monitoring
Western blot	Human immunodeficiency virus

SKELETAL SYSTEM

Alkaline phosphatase (ALP)	Bone disorders
Antinuclear antibody (ANA)	Systemic lupus erythematosus/collagen disorders
Calcium (Ca)	Bone disorders
Erythrocyte sedimentation rate (ESR)	Inflammation
Fluorescent antinuclear antibody (FANA)	Systemic lupus erythematosus/collagen disorders
Phosphorus (P)	Skeletal disorders
Rheumatoid arthritis (RA)	Rheumatoid arthritis
Uric acid	Gout
Vitamin D	Calcium absorption

MUSCULAR SYSTEM

Creatine kinase [CK(CPK)]	Muscle damage
Creatine kinase isoenzymes (CK-MM)	Muscle damage
Lactic acid	Muscle disorders
Magnesium (Mg)	Musculoskeletal disorders
Myoglobin	Muscle damage
Potassium (K)	Muscle function

Continued

NERVOUS SYSTEM	
Creatine kinase isoenzymes (CK-BB)	Brain damage
Cerebral spinal fluid (CSF) (cell count, glucose, protein, culture)	Neurological disorders or meningitis
Drug screening	Therapeutic drug monitoring or drug abuse
Lead	Neurological function
Lithium (Li)	Antidepressant drug monitoring

RESPIRATORY SYSTEM	
Arterial blood gases (ABGs)	Acid-base balance
Cold agglutinins	Atypical pneumonia
Complete blood count (CBC)	Pneumonia
Electrolytes (Lytes)	Acid-base balance
Gram stain	Microbial infection
Throat and sputum cultures	Bacterial infection

DIGESTIVE SYSTEM	
Alanine aminotransferase [ALT(SGPT)]	Liver disorders
Albumin	Malnutrition or liver disorders
Alcohol	Intoxication/liver function
Alkaline phosphatase (ALP)	Liver disorders
Ammonia	Severe liver disorders
Amylase	Pancreatitis
Anti–hepatitis B surface antigen	Immunity to hepatitis B
Anti–hepatitis C virus	Viral hepatitis
Aspartate aminotransferase [AST(SGOT)]	Liver disorders
Bilirubin	Liver disorders
Carcinoembryonic antigen (CEA)	Carcinoma detection and monitoring
Complete blood count (CBC)	Appendicitis, peritonitis, or other infection
Gamma-glutamyltransferase (GGT)	Early liver disorders
Gastrin	Gastric malignancy
Hepatitis A, B, and C immunoassays	Hepatitis A, B, and C screening
Lactate dehydrogenase [LD(LDH)]	Liver disorders
Lipase	Pancreatitis
Occult blood	Gastrointestinal bleeding or intestinal malignancy
Stool culture	Pathogenic bacteria
Total protein (TP)	Liver disorders

URINARY SYSTEM	
Albumin	Kidney disorders
Ammonia	Hepatic encephalopathy
Antistreptolysin O (ASO) titer	Acute glomerulonephritis
Blood urea nitrogen (BUN)	Kidney disorders
Creatinine	Kidney disorders
Creatinine clearance	Glomerular filtration
Electrolytes (Lytes)	Fluid and electrolyte balance

URINARY SYSTEM—cont'd

Osmolality	Fluid and electrolyte balance
Routine Urinalysis	Renal or metabolic disorders
Total protein (TP)	Kidney disorders
Uric acid	Kidney disorders
Urine culture	Bacterial infection

ENDOCRINE SYSTEM

Adrenocorticotropic hormone (ACTH)	Adrenal and pituitary gland function
Aldosterone	Adrenal function
Antidiuretic hormone (ADH)	Pituitary function
Calcium (Ca)	Parathyroid function
Cortisol	Adrenal cortex function
Glucose	Hypoglycemia or diabetes mellitus
Glucose tolerance test (GTT)	Hypoglycemia or diabetes mellitus
Growth hormone (GH)	Pituitary gland function
Insulin	Glucose metabolism and pancreatic function
Parathyroid hormone (PTH)	Parathyroid function
Phosphorus (P)	Endocrine disorders
Testosterone	Testicular function
Thyroid function (T3, T4, TSH) studies	Thyroid function

REPRODUCTIVE SYSTEM

Acid phosphatase	Prostate cancer
Estradiol, estriol, and estrogen	Ovarian or placental function
Fluorescent treponemal antibody–absorbed (FTA-ABS)	Syphilis
Genital culture	Microbial infection
Gram stain	Microbial infection
Human chorionic gonadotropin (Beta HCG)	Pregnancy
Pap smear (PAP)	Cervical or vaginal carcinoma
Prostate-specific antigen (PSA)	Prostatic cancer
Prostatic acid phosphatase (PAP)	Prostatic cancer
Rapid plasma reagin (RPR)	Syphilis
Rubella titer	Immunity to German measles
Semen analysis	Infertility or effectiveness of vasectomy
Toxoplasma antibody screening	Toxoplasma infection
Vaginal wet prep	Fungal infection
Venereal Disease Research Laboratory (VDRL)	Syphilis

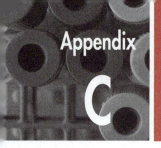

Answer Keys to Review Questions and Situation Exercises

Unit 1

ANSWERS TO SAFETY SITUATIONS EXERCISE

1. **a.** Yes, if there is enough urine to perform the test.
   b. The outsides of the tubes must be disinfected with a 1:10 dilution of sodium hypochlorite (bleach) and the labels replaced.
   c. The urine and blood specimens should have been sent in separate properly labeled plastic sealable biohazard bags.
   d. Both specimens could possibly be rejected by the laboratory because of contamination.

2. **a.** Immediately rinse the blood from the puncture site and report the incident to a supervisor.
   b. HBV, HCV, and HIV
   c. PPE will be started if the source patient tests positive for HIV or HBV.
   d. Thorough instruction on the use of the safety device must take place before using any device as each is a little different.

ANSWERS TO REVIEW QUESTIONS

1. D
2. B
3. D
4. C
5. C
6. B
7. A
8. D
9. A
10. D

Unit 2

ANSWERS TO REVIEW QUESTIONS

1. D
2. D
3. C
4. B
5. A
6. C
7. A
8. A
9. B
10. D

Unit 3

ANSWERS TO VENIPUNCTURE SITUATIONS EXERCISE

1. **a.** Not acceptable. The patient may become faint or dizzy during the procedure and collapse on the floor.
   b. Acceptable. The tourniquet would be applied too long if the equipment was not assembled first.
   c. Not acceptable. This will cause hemoconcentration of the specimen.
   d. Acceptable. This provides maximum sterility at the actual puncture site.
   e. Not acceptable. This enlarges the puncture hole possibly causing a hematoma.

2. **a.** A hematoma: Bending the patient's arm when applying pressure.
   b. Petechiae: Leaving the tourniquet on too tightly for too long.
   c. A patient to choke: Allowing the patient to have gum, a thermometer, or other item in his or her mouth while performing venipuncture.
   d. Blood to stop flowing when a tube is changed: The needle has moved either through the vein or out of the vein.
   e. Blood drops on a patient's slacks when the needle is removed: Failure to remove the last tube from the holder before removing the needle

ANSWER TO REVIEW QUESTIONS

1. C
2. B
3. A
4. D
5. A
6. B
7. B
8. C
9. C
10. A

Unit 4

ANSWERS TO VENIPUNCTURE COMPLICATION SITUATIONS EXERCISE

1. Attach temporary identification to the patient. Use a commercial blood bank identification system.

2. Request another blood collector to collect the PT.

3. **a.** 2
   b. X
   c. 1

4. 2.7 mL in the light blue stopper tube, 2.0 mL in the lavender stopper tube, 2.3 mL in the red stopper tube

5. **a.** Collapsed vein
   b. Use smaller evacuated tubes. Use a syringe.

6. **a.** Blood is leaking out of the vein into the tissue.
   b. Remove the needle and apply pressure.
   c. Use a 23-gauge needle with a syringe or butterfly.

7. a. The specimen contained small clots.
   b. The blood collector was busy with the patient and did not mix the specimen.
   c. Yes. Use one hand to mix the specimen as soon as the patient's head is lowered.

8. Inadequate pressure is being applied to the site. These patients are often taking anticoagulants and require additional pressure.

9. a. The specimen was hemolyzed.
   b. Do not leave the tourniquet on for more than 1 minute.

   Use a smaller evacuated tube.
   Avoid mixing the sample.
   If the blood is collected in a syringe, immediately transfer it to the evacuated tube.

10. a. The skin may be thin and bruised when applying a tourniquet. A blood pressure cuff may be used. A bandage may take off a layer of skin when being removed.
   b. Partial draw or small volume tubes and a winged blood collection set (butterfly) with a 23-gauge needle
   c. Incompletely filled light blue stopper tube.
   d. Difficulty in locating and anchoring veins; increased danger of hematoma formation; prone to bruising; increased risk of infection.
   e. Visually confirm that the puncture site has stopped bleeding and apply a self-adhering bandage rather than an adhesive bandage.

11. a. Possible nerve damage
   b. A 15 degree angle with the bevel up. The median cubital vein is the vein of choice. The basilic vein is the last choice and a needle angle of greater than 30 degrees should never be employed.
   c. Extensive probing may hemolyze the specimen; therefore, causing the laboratory to reject the specimen.

ANSWERS TO REVIEW QUESTIONS
   1. C
   2. A
   3. C
   4. D
   5. D
   6. C
   7. B
   8. D
   9. A
   10. D

Unit 5

ANSWERS TO SPECIAL VENIPUNCTURE COLLECTION EXERCISE

1. Has the patient been fasting for 12 hours?

2. Yes, the patient may be bleeding internally and must be monitored.

3. Check to be sure the patient is fasting. Draw the fasting specimen. Instruct the patient to eat a full breakfast and return exactly 2 hours after completing breakfast. Draw the 2-hour specimen.

4. Notify the supervisor or physician about the vomiting. If the physician cannot be reached in time, collect the 3-hour specimen and note the vomiting on the requisition.

5. Cortisol levels should be drawn between 0800 and 1000. Collect the specimen before the patient goes to physical therapy.

6. No. The 0800 request would be the trough level, and the 1200 request could be the peak level.

7. Yes. The patient needs to be started on antibiotics.

8. a. Aseptic technique was not followed. One set was collected in the wrong tube.
   b. The anticoagulant in the lavender stopper tube killed the bacteria.

9. The ammonia level will be decreased because the specimen was not chilled immediately. The cold agglutinin will be decreased because it was not kept warm. The CBC will be unaffected.

10. a. 1. How do you know you collected blood from the right person?
       2. How did you disinfect the person's arm?
       3. How do you know the specimen you drew from this patient did not get mixed up with another specimen?
   b. 1. The blood collector explains the appropriate identification procedure and identifies a witness.
       2. The blood collector explains the use of cleansing agents other than alcohol.
       3. The blood collector explains the chain of custody procedure and produces it as documentation.

ANSWERS TO REVIEW QUESTIONS

1. C
2. C
3. B
4. B
5. TRUE
6. C
7. C
8. B
9. D
10. C

Unit 6

ANSWERS TO DERMAL PUNCTURE COLLECTION EXERCISE

1. a. The alcohol should be allowed to dry and the first drop wiped away. Failure to let the alcohol dry on the puncture site produces hemolysis.
   b. Scraping the skin to collect blood flowing down the finger will cause hemolysis.
   c. Yes. If blood from a second puncture is added to the first tube, hemolysis and microclots may occur.

2. a. Confirm that the alcohol is completely dry.
   b. Confirm that the puncture is made across the finger or heel print. Blood from punctures aligned with the fingerprint does not form rounded drops.

    c. Failure to firmly press the puncture device on the site does not cause a deep enough puncture to produce a rounded drop.

    d. Continual pressure to the area around the puncture site decreases the flow of blood to the puncture.

3. a. Yes

    b. The lavender Microtainer should be collected first because platelets immediately begin adhering to the puncture site.

ANSWERS TO REVIEW QUESTIONS

  1. C
  2. A
  3. B
  4. B
  5. D
  6. B
  7. C
  8. A
  9. A
10. B

Unit 7

ANSWERS TO POINT-OF-CARE EXERCISES

1. a. Rerun the QC—repeat the finger stick and repeat the glucose test.

    b. Insufficent specimen applied to the testing strip; defective testing strip; instrument not correctly calibrated.

2. a. No

    b. Rerun the QC; test on a new abnormal high control.

    c. Outdated reagent test strip; discolored reagent test strip; contaminated test strip; test strips and analyzer code number don't match; control is outdated or contaminated.

ANSWERS TO REVIEW QUESTIONS

  1. C
  2. B
  3. D
  4. B
  5. A
  6. B
  7. B
  8. D
  9. B
10. D

Unit 8

ANSWERS TO INTRAVENOUS AND CVCs EXERCISE

1. **a.** 5 syringes
   b. 4 syringes
   c. An evacuated tube holder

2. **a.** Pulling the plunger of the syringe too rapidly.
   b. Forcing blood from the syringe into an evacuated tube.

3. **a.** The appearance of blood in the hub of a syringe needle or the small chamber of a catheter. Flashback indicates you have successfully entered the vein.
   b. Syringes filled with sterile saline that are used to prime collection equipment such as a stopcock. Syringes used to clear a line prior to collecting blood or infusing a different substance into a line that has already been infusing a medication or treatment. Syringes used to clear a line following blood collection to avoid occlusion of the line by allowing blood to clot in the line.

ANSWERS TO REVIEW QUESTIONS

1. B
2. C
3. B
4. B
5. A
6. D
7. B
8. C
9. A
10. A

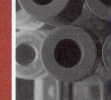

Index

Page numbers followed by "f" denote figures; "b" denote boxes; and "t" denote tables